HEALING the BROKEN BRAIN

"An insightful and comprehensive how-to guide to surviving stroke."

— **Mehmet Oz, M.D.,** professor of surgery, NewYork-Presbyterian/
Columbia University Medical Center

"A groundbreaking guide for the prevention and treatment of stroke."

— **Daniel Amen, M.D.,** *New York Times* best-selling author of
The Brain Warrior's Way

"As the mother of a child who suffered a life-threatening brain injury, I
know the power of combining hope with science in healing broken brains.
With this book, Mike and David have provided that combination to all
stroke survivors and the family members who believe in them."

— **JJ Virgin,** *New York Times* best-selling author of *Miracle Mindset*

"Dr. Mike and his brother David reveal a profound truth in this incredible
book: spiritual growth and faith are required when faced with life's most
difficult roadblocks."

— **Gabrielle Bernstein,** #1 *New York Times* best-selling author of
The Universe Has Your Back

"Patience, mindfulness, and optimism are all tools needed in the recovery
journey from a stroke. Dr. Mike Dow and his brother do an amazing job
delivering a healthy dose of inspiration and insight.
A must read for survivors and caregivers!"

— **Dr. Susan Albers,** *New York Times* best-selling author of *50 Ways to
Soothe Yourself Without Food, Eating Mindfully,* and *Eat.Q.*

"This book should be required reading for all stroke survivors and the people who love them."

— **Tana Amen, B.S.N., R.N.,** *New York Times* best-selling author of *The Omni Diet*

"This thorough and compassionate guide for families and survivors will provide relief, comfort, and wisdom to all who read it."

— **Andrea Pennington, M.D., C.Ac.,** best-selling author of *Daily Compassion Meditation*

"As the family member of a stroke survivor, I know it takes a village of doctors to optimize recovery. Mike and David have delivered this village to all stroke survivors and their families through this life-changing book."

— **Allison Arthur, M.D.,** Mayo Clinic-trained physician and co-owner of Sand Lake Dermatology Center

HEALING the
BROKEN BRAIN

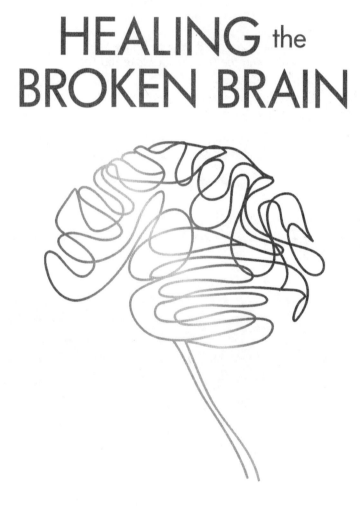

ALSO BY DR. MIKE DOW

*The Brain Fog Fix: Reclaim Your Focus, Memory,
and Joy in Just 3 Weeks*

*Diet Rehab: 28 Days to Finally Stop
Craving the Foods That Make You Fat*

ALSO BY DAVID DOW

Brain Attack: My Journey of Recovery from Stroke and Aphasia

HEALING the BROKEN BRAIN

LEADING EXPERTS ANSWER
100 QUESTIONS
ABOUT STROKE RECOVERY

Dr. Mike Dow
& David Dow
with Megan Sutton, CCC-SLP

HAY HOUSE, INC.
Carlsbad, California • New York City
London • Sydney • Johannesburg
Vancouver • New Delhi

Published and distributed in the United States by: Hay House, Inc.: www
.hayhouse.com® • *Published and distributed in Australia by:* Hay House Australia Pty.
Ltd.: www.hayhouse.com.au • *Published and distributed in the United Kingdom by:*
Hay House UK, Ltd.: www.hayhouse.co.uk • *Published and distributed in the Republic
of South Africa by:* Hay House SA (Pty), Ltd.: www.hayhouse.co.za • *Distributed in
Canada by:* Raincoast Books: www.raincoast.com • *Published in India by:* Hay House
Publishers India: www.hayhouse.co.in

Cover Designer: Tricia Breidenthal • *Interior design:* Pamela Homan • *Indexer:* Jay Kreider
MRI image and photo of young David Dow in ICU on page xxi: Carol Dow-Richards
Photo of adult David Dow on page xxi: Barbara Baie

Library of Congress Cataloging-in-Publication Data

Names: Dow, Mike, author. | Dow, David, author. | Sutton, Megan, author.
Title: Healing the broken brain : leading experts answer 100 questions about stroke recovery / Dr.
Mike Dow and David Dow, with Megan Sutton, CCC-SLP.
Description: Carlsbad, California : Hay House, Inc., [2017]
Identifiers: LCCN 2016046665 | ISBN 9781401952655 (paperback)
Subjects: LCSH: Cerebrovascular disease--Treatment. | Cerebrovascular disease--Miscellanea. | BI-
SAC: HEALTH & FITNESS / Diseases / Nervous System (incl. Brain). | HEALTH & FITNESS / General.
| HEALTH & FITNESS / Diseases / General.
Classification: LCC RC388.5 .D69 2017 | DDC 616.8/1--dc23 LC record available at https://lccn.
loc.gov/2016046665

Tradepaper ISBN: 978-1-4019-5265-5

10 9 8 7 6 5 4 3 2 1
1st edition, May 2017

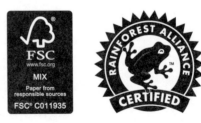

CONTENTS

"In the treatment of brain injury the story starts out darkly. The patient is a shadow: damaged, frightened, and withdrawn. But as physicians, therapists, and family connect, hope grows anew, recovery begins, and pages turn. And it is an appreciation of the simplest parts of ourselves, something simpler than we could ever believe, that begins personal recovery on the neurorehabilitation unit. When we can make these shadows dance, that is the art of brain repair."

— Dr. Tom Carmichael

INTRODUCTION

Moments that drastically change your life tend to come out of nowhere. They're like unexpected and unwanted guests. You: the unprepared and unwilling host. As you're left blindsided and bewildered, you are immediately thrust into a new reality and must come to terms with a "new normal" whether you like it or not. My family had one of those days 20 years ago when my brother, David, had a massive stroke. He was just 10 years old.

If you're reading this book, it probably means you or someone you love has had a stroke. You or your loved one is now a stroke survivor. You can probably relate to the feelings of confusion that my brother and family felt when we were dealing with the initial onslaught of information about stroke. It's hard to fully comprehend everything being said by the team of specialists flooding your hospital room— especially if you happen to be a stroke survivor with newly impaired language skills.

I remember walking down a depressing hospital hallway with my mom as she cried, telling me that David had something called aphasia. As a 15-year-old, I'd never heard that word before. To me, this confusing word felt like he had yet *another* problem on top of the stroke. People kept saying this word with the same tone you might use if you were saying a phrase like "stage-four cancer."

Like many of you, I have my own traumatic memories. I saw my mom lose it in a department store as she was too exhausted to pick out a new shirt after she had run out of clean clothes, having practically lived at the hospital. I remember that feeling of dread in my stomach when I realized that something had changed and life would never go back to the way it was before.

This is our family's story, but I know you have your own personal experience. Like snowflakes, each stroke is unique. Different parts of the brain affect different language skills, body parts, behavior, mood, and even who we are. Doctors will sum up this frightening mixed bag you've been handed with medical terms and acronyms that will sound like a foreign language. And as human beings, the unfamiliar and unknown is inherently scarier than challenges or situations we understand. Most experts just don't have the time to fully educate you on everything you need to know in the 10 minutes they have before they need to get ready for their next patient. And, that next patient needs their help as much as you do. But that doesn't change the fact that you're still left wanting more.

Trust me—there's *a lot* to learn. Especially when you're dealing with the part of your body that makes you who you are and is involved in every decision and every move you make: your brain. One important lesson my brother and mom learned as survivor and advocate was this: Being passive has no place in stroke recovery. You have to educate yourself, ask questions, do more than the minimum, and become a fighter.

My brother fought for his recovery every day. There were moments of hopelessness, frustration, and sadness. I know mourning his old life and coming to terms with his new normal was a seemingly unbearable experience at times. This pained me so much that I often coped by just trying not to think about my brother's condition. After all, I was attempting to be a normal kid in high school. It was just too hard. As I lay in my bed in our home, and as he lay in his in a children's hospital, I knew we were both wishing for the same thing: to be "normal" again and for everything to just go back to the way it was. How do you make sense of something so painful? How can you keep the faith that good things happen in the world, when everything feels so bleak?

Well, let me tell you a story about my brother that just may help break up a few of the clouds hanging over you today. David recently had an appointment with a new neurologist. The doctor had my brother's brain scans in hand when David walked into his office for the first time.

"You're David Dow?!" he said. "You can't possibly be! You shouldn't even be *walking* into my office!"

With a look of pure awe on his face, this doctor—who was supposed to be the one telling *him* what is and isn't possible—just couldn't believe what he was witnessing. You see, my brother's stroke was massive. Looking at his brain scan, you could see that the entire left side was affected.

How did my brother beat the odds and exceed all the doctors' expectations? How did David become the one showing this doctor what was possible? One step, one letter, one sound, one movement, one session, one challenge, and one day at a time—for 20 years. His therapy wasn't confined to hospitals, because for David and all stroke survivors, recovery fills every day and every moment of life after the stroke occurs.

But I can confidently say that dark skies do give way to sunshine. David is not in a nursing home as they told us he would be. He lives an independent and active life. He drives. He's in a relationship. He has friends. He travels. But to achieve the goals that seemed impossible, my brother and my family had to find and apply the most groundbreaking research. Sometimes, this meant seeking a second or third opinion. It meant making a case with our health insurance company and fighting for more therapy sessions. And after we educated ourselves, David was the one who had to do the work—the painful, difficult, and scary work of recovering.

After three doctors insisted that David's case was inoperable, we sought out the opinion of one of the top neurosurgeons in the country. Not operating meant that the extremely rare brain disease that caused the stroke would likely lead to more strokes until David was unable to move at all—or until he was dead. This gifted surgeon performed two difficult, major reconstructive brain surgeries on David. David hasn't had another stroke since.

David went through a course of constraint therapy, which involves restraining the good limb to force the affected limb to do all the work. Of course, this can be frustrating when a person painstakingly spends minutes trying to take a bite of dinner with a hand that's not getting sufficient signals from the brain. Picture boards helped David communicate when he was unable to utter a sound. Slowly, sounds became words, and those became phrases, which eventually became sentences.

Doctors told us David had up to six months to recover. After that, we were told, progress would come to a screeching halt. That was the prevalent belief in the 1990s. Unfortunately, stroke survivors are still sometimes told this today. Don't believe this myth. Hope creates a state of optimism that can take you just a little bit further, whereas pessimism creates a self-fulfilling state associated with depression and inaction. It's possible that you will be more recovered next month than you are this month, and it's probable that you will be more recovered next year than you are this year. My mom knew the power of what we tell ourselves. She would lie next to David in his hospital bed and share positive thoughts: "I am getting better. I am getting stronger. I will recover." Her words became his beliefs, which became his actions.

This optimism paid off. Today, David gets on stages and gives entire speeches to stroke survivors—something he never could have done six months after his stroke. I look forward to the day when experimental treatments like stem cell therapy help David take his recovery to the next level. I can't wait for the day I see him writing with his right hand again. I hope all survivors will benefit from the clinical trials that are now taking place.

But as we all look forward to new treatments in the future, we also have to work with the tools we have now and deal with today's changes in the health-care system. A stroke survivor today will not receive the number of hours of insurance-funded therapy my brother received decades ago. The limited hours of therapy a stroke survivor gets today are, of course, helpful, but, they probably won't get the person to where he or she would ultimately like to be. Other things have changed for the better. Technology can pick up where health insurance leaves off. In fact, our co-writer, Megan Sutton, is the creator of the Tactus Therapy apps, which utilize clinically proven speech therapy principles in exercises to do at home on a tablet or phone. This technology wasn't available 20 years ago, when it would have been extremely useful to David, but these apps are something my mom and brother highly recommend to members of their aphasia support organization.

What does all this mean? It means your true therapy has only just begun when you finish your last formal session of speech, occupational, or physical therapy at the hospital. Your *life* becomes the therapy.

What will you do with it? Will you isolate yourself in front of the TV all day? Will you let your frustration make you give up and throw in the towel? Or will you decide to take a few more steps today than you did yesterday? Will you use your speech therapy app for another 15 minutes? Will you reach out to old friends while making new ones? Will you go out in public and make your best effort, even when it feels hard to do so? These everyday decisions are important because when it comes to the brain, it's use it or lose it. Figure out simple ways you can use yours today. Every conversation you have is now speech therapy. Every step you take is physical therapy.

Everything you do that challenges you is now therapy because these activities challenge your brain, and by doing so, your brain has the ability to change itself. You'll hear about this concept of brain regrowth and rewiring—called neuroplasticity—over and over again throughout this book. Decades ago, scientists believed that the brain stops growing in early childhood. But we now know the human brain has the power to create new brain cells throughout an entire lifetime—as long as it's properly challenged. What this means for stroke survivors is that while there is usually more rapid recovery in the months following a stroke, it's possible to continue to make gains for years. So whether a stroke occurs at 10 or 70, there is an opportunity to rewire and regrow cells that can help you to reach the next level of your recovery.

My brother and I were called to write this book in order to become guides for those of you who would like to join us. We know what it's like to be confused and alone. We know you have questions—lots of them. So our goal here is to provide you with a road map. This book is packed with information from the leading experts in stroke recovery. We believe that it won't just educate you; it will also provide you with hope for what's possible for you or your loved one. My brother's story will infuse you with a shot of faith when you need it most. You'll be equipped with the knowledge of what to do as well as some of the best ways to execute the next steps.

I also hope that somewhere down the line there will be some purpose, meaning, and sense-making that emerges for you personally. At 15 I never could have predicted that the compassion and emotional depth I gained from David's journey would somehow blossom into a deep desire to help others. It started with me doing part-time volunteer work at a Ronald McDonald House, one of the places that housed my family when my brother was sick. Then it blossomed into a full-time career and what I now know is, for me, a calling. I got a master's and doctorate degree in psychology. I became obsessed with the integrative strategies that help the brain heal itself, such as taking the omega-3 supplements my physician father made my brother take daily at a time when many people in mainstream medicine regarded them as snake oil and were touting low-fat diets for overall health. In actuality, the fatty acids found in fish oil act as the building blocks for your brain's cells and are crucial to neuroplasticity, and diets higher in healthy fats may be better for the brain than low-fat ones. These are just some of many tools that can help your brain heal. I continue to seek out the newest developments in mental health, psychopharmacology, nutrition, exercise, experimental treatments, mindfulness, and even spirituality for their profound abilities to change the brain.

These forward-thinking principles formed the foundation of my book *The Brain Fog Fix,* which, looking back, grew out of my personal belief in the brain's incredible power to heal itself as well as our uniquely human capacity to heal ourselves. While that book wasn't written specifically for stroke survivors, many of the principles described inside are universal. The modified Mediterranean diet I recommend—which helps a normal, aging brain retain its edge and prevents dementia—is the same diet that can help stroke survivors heal. Cognitive behavioral strategies don't just help a person deal with a breakup; they also help a stroke survivor remain resilient through a frustrating day of speech therapy. It's not just stroke survivors who desperately want a better brain. We all do. And I believe this universal desire is what made *The Brain Fog Fix* a bestseller. As the quote goes,

"When God closes a door, he opens a window." It turns out my window led me down an unexpected path with an outcome I never could have predicted.

And I certainly never would have predicted that my brother and mom would go on to form Aphasia Recovery Connection, a nonprofit that helps other stroke survivors, and make it their mission in life. They now bring stroke survivors and their families together for support—online, on cruises, and in a residential boot camp. The lemonade you make from *your* lemons may be as simple as making new friends or taking the time to appreciate small victories and life's simple joys. Maybe the experience you've been through will come in handy when a friend goes through a similar experience and needs someone to talk to on a dark day. Maybe you'll have a new perspective on life as you realize what's truly important in this world.

Let me tell you a little bit about how we wrote this book. David and I started by interviewing world-class experts. Hours of interviews were condensed into a vital and easy-to-understand manual for anyone who is fighting for their own stroke recovery or supporting the recovery of someone they love.

This book is made up of 100 questions we knew stroke survivors and their families would want answered. David asked our experts questions that came from real stroke survivors. The questions start out basic but then get more specific as we tackle different areas of recovery. For stroke survivors still struggling with reading comprehension or for family members who are too tired to read long passages of information, we've summarized the takeaway points in simple language at the end of each chapter. Medical words are in *italics* so you can learn what they mean or look up more information. Key concepts are **bolded** for quick scanning. Also, this book is available in audiobook format for anyone with vision or reading-comprehension difficulties. In the audiobook you'll also get to hear David's voice and my voice as we walk you through this journey.

In Part I, we look at some of the basics of what a stroke is and what happens when you have one. Top doctors guide you through the medical terminology and let you know what to expect. In Part II, we talk to some of the top rehabilitation experts to find out what goes wrong with both the body and the brain after a stroke. These therapists offer advice on how to improve your walking, your use of arms and hands, your cognition, and your communication, as well as how to make the most of your therapy. In Part III, we continue with expert advice for recovery, but we focus on your life as a whole rather than just your physical body. Finding purpose, motivation, and overall health will get you back into living, no matter where you are in your rehab. Finally, in Part IV, we offer advice for caregivers. Our experts have also shared their insight into what's coming in the field of stroke recovery, so you'll know what you can look forward to in the future. There are also helpful resources in the back of the book so you can continue your recovery.

Throughout this book, you'll see quotes from David that share his experiences. You'll see boxes with practical tips from our co-writer, Megan. In addition to creating the Tactus Therapy apps and advocating for stroke survivors, she's one of the most respected speech therapists in the recovery field. I've also offered my expertise throughout, giving you exercises and advice to help you heal. Together, we hope this book will serve as your Stroke Recovery 101.

Maybe you're reading this book in a hospital room like the one in which my brother and family spent so many hours. Maybe you're sitting in the waiting room while your husband finishes his speech therapy. Maybe something in David's story will inspire you to work a little harder today, and maybe today will be the day you take your first few steps or get a little more movement in your hand. Maybe you'll realize that while it's okay to be sad, you are the only one who can make the decision not to give up—even on the days when you feel absolutely alone in this world. Wherever you are in your recovery journey, David and I hope that this book will help you understand that you are not alone. We hope that after reading it, you too will do everything in your power to heal your broken brain.

A NOTE FROM DAVID
TO STROKE SURVIVORS

When I was little, my life was a piece of cake. I loved to read and play soccer and hang out with my friends. I enjoyed playing the bells at church each Sunday. And I actually looked forward to school. My goal in life was to become a doctor like my dad, and I hoped to have a large family of my own someday. It seemed I was on the right track to achieve those goals—until my life took a turn for the worse.

It was Christmas of 1994, and I was 10 years old. After we finished opening our presents, my grandparents told me and Mike that they had one last special gift for us. They gave us clues about what the surprise was: a golden lion, an emerald city, Greek gods, a large pyramid with cool hieroglyphics inside. Mike guessed it. The surprise was a family vacation to Las Vegas that spring! I was so excited. It was going to be a trip that we'd never forget. Unfortunately, that turned out to be all too true, and our lives would never be the same.

March came and we were off to Vegas. We were supposed to go hiking in the canyons, but I started to have flu-like symptoms. My mom and I stayed behind while the others headed out, and I lay down to rest. When I woke up, I could no longer talk and my right side was dragging like a dead fish. I was having a stroke.

I don't remember much about the next few weeks. I didn't understand what was going on and couldn't understand what people were saying. It was like waking up in a country where you don't speak the language. I was hooked up to machines and had tubes in my arms, and people kept sticking needles into me. The doctors ran tests and eventually discovered that I had a rare vascular abnormality called *Moyamoya disease*, which is what caused the stroke. I lived in the hospital for nearly three months. I couldn't speak or understand because of a condition called global aphasia, and I lost the use of the entire right side of my body. Nearly all of the left side of my brain was damaged.

One doctor recommended that my parents move me to a nursing home for the rest of my life. He said that it would be best for everyone since I would be permanently disabled. After staying with me for the first 10 days, my family had to go back home to Ohio. They had to get back to work and school. But my mom didn't go. She stayed by my side in the hospital. I knew she felt hopeless—and desperate for help. She was asking anyone she could for advice, but the doctors came in and out so quickly that it was hard to get any answers. She begged one doctor to tell her what he would do if I were his family member. He gave her this advice: "Stimulate, stimulate, stimulate—and fight!"

So we became fighters. It wasn't easy. I had to learn how to walk again. I had to learn how to talk again. I could use only one hand. Speech therapy taught me the tools and techniques to communicate in other ways. In the beginning, the progress was slow. I used word and image boards so I could point to what I needed. I had to learn simple words like *yes* and *no*. I got confused hearing simple questions like "Do you want some water?" Then I started to relearn single words to communicate what I needed: *food, sleep, TV*. Physical therapy helped me with my legs, allowing me to go from using a wheelchair to walking between parallel bars to using a cane. I had to learn how to write with my nondominant left hand in occupational therapy. My three-day trip to Las Vegas ended up being nearly three months of inpatient rehab. I continued outpatient therapy and rehabilitation for nearly 15 years.

Fast-forward to today. I can walk. I can talk. I can drive. I have many *abilities*. Things aren't as easy as before, but I live independently and try to have a normal life. I enjoy traveling, watching movies, and listening to podcasts. At times during my recovery, I was unsure if I'd ever be able to live on my own. But I have improved and adapted. Getting out of my comfort zone has helped my recovery, but it hasn't always been easy. Sometimes other people do not understand me.

Occasionally, people have been cruel. In the beginning, some people thought I was drunk or dumb because of my aphasia. I hated that.

Now I travel on my own. I've visited foreign countries and figured out how to get around by myself. My independence and my ability to book complex itineraries are evidence of my recovery.

Don't get me wrong. Many things are still an issue for me, such as my *agraphia* (writing difficulty), so I find tools to help me. For example, I used speech-to-text software to help me write this introduction. I have difficulty putting sentences together and editing, so I use that software to play back the words in order to find places where something's not right. I can hear—but not always see—what needs to be changed.

I tend to sleep a lot because the pathways in my damaged brain get overloaded. I get severe back and body pain from overworking my left side, which I still favor. I still have aphasia, and it's more pronounced when I am stressed or tired. However, all of those *disabilities* do not stop me from living my life. And yours shouldn't stop you.

Whatever stage of stroke recovery you are in, please know that you are not alone. I've been there, and so have millions of others. I've felt hopeless. I've felt lonely. I've felt scared, frustrated, confused, and angry. All stroke survivors have. But there's a reason they call us survivors. We're fighters—not victims.

On the last night of my hospital stay, my doctor gave me a watch as a going-away gift. When I looked at the face of it, I saw it had a soldier on it. She said, "Be a fighter." I wore that watch to remind me that I was in a battle. I was a fighter. I needed a battle plan. And so do you.

This book is meant to help you in your fight. Use it as a guide to help you get through the dark times when you don't know what to do next. My brother and I talked to the top experts in the field of stroke recovery to ask questions on your behalf. The medical professionals in these chapters are speaking directly to you—the stroke survivor or family member. But unlike voices that fade away, this advice is kept safe for you on these pages to read and reread when you need it. Stroke recovery is a marathon, not a sprint. You'll need different tools at each stage of the race.

The good news is that my life is still on the right track. It's just a different track than the one I imagined as a child. There's purpose in my life. I truly believe that somehow this is where I belonged the whole time: helping others find hope and see possibilities. Now I want to help *you* find the ways to achieve your highest potential and enjoy life. From the bottom of my heart, I believe that we can do this—together!

Remember to take your recovery one day at time. There is so much to learn and so much to do. It can be overwhelming. Sometimes you'll feel like you just don't know where to turn.

I spent many years feeling hopelessness and despair. Recovery is hard. But what I learned is that if I took tiny steps and built on that, I made progress. It was very slow and the progress was almost unnoticeable, but it was happening. At the same time, I was learning techniques that would help me adapt to—rather than overcome—my paralysis and communication difficulties.

Today, I am a founding board member of the Aphasia Recovery Connection, a nonprofit that works to help families dealing with the language difficulties I have struggled with. We have the world's largest support group for people with aphasia, do aphasia cruises (which I organize), and run an Aphasia University Boot Camp in Las Vegas. You can learn more about our nonprofit at the end of this book.

I hope you find the book helpful. Take notes. Structure time to learn and work on recovery. Practice what you do well and build on it. Ask for help. Create healthy habits. Take up new hobbies. Get to know other stroke survivors by attending support groups in your local area or on Facebook. Connect. Maybe I'll get to meet you at an Aphasia Recovery Connection event someday. Even if you don't make a full recovery back to your prestroke self (I didn't), aim for your own personal, optimal recovery—whatever that looks like for you. I hope that you too will have a recovery story with some silver linings.

Stay positive! I got through it, and I know you can too.

Warmly,
David

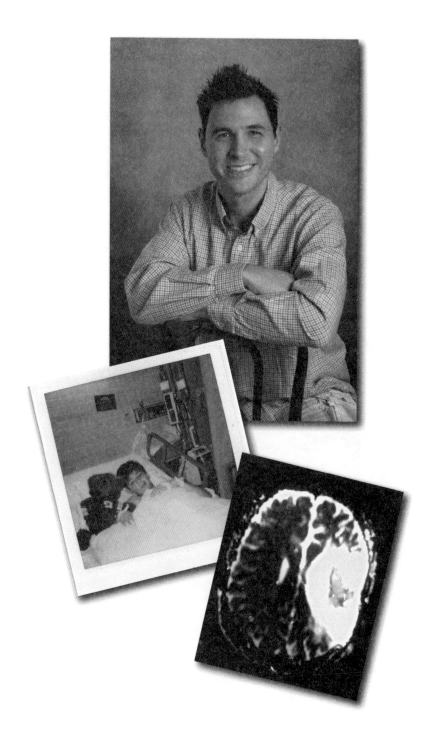

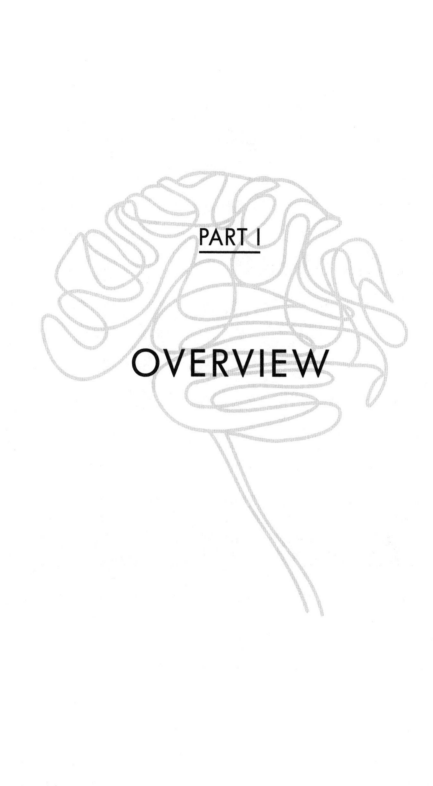

PART I

OVERVIEW

CHAPTER 1

UNDERSTANDING STROKE

Nearly everyone has heard of a stroke, and most people know someone who has had one. To help you better understand what a stroke really is, why strokes occur, and who is likely to have one, we asked the experts to explain. Dr. Elliot Roth is the chairman of the Department of Physical Medicine and Rehabilitation at Northwestern University and the medical director of the Patient Recovery Unit at the Rehabilitation Institute of Chicago. Dr. David Chiu is a neurologist and the medical director of the stroke center at Houston Methodist Hospital. They are both physicians and researchers at leading hospitals in the treatment of stroke, and they answer your questions about what happens during a stroke and how to prevent one from happening again.

1. What is a stroke?

Author's note: A stroke is a disruption of blood flow in the brain. Like the rest of our body, the brain depends on a network of blood vessels to carry oxygen and nutrients to the cells. When those vessels become blocked or damaged, part of the brain doesn't receive the oxygen it needs. When brain cells are impaired or killed, the function in the part of the body those cells control is compromised—making the body part weak, paralyzed, or uncoordinated.

3

Because of the way the brain is organized, damage to one side of the brain affects the *opposite* side of the body (e.g., a stroke affecting the *right* side of the brain may impair the use of the *left* arm and leg). After a stroke, a stroke survivor will experience an array of effects on the mind and body, the number and severity depending on where, how much of, and how long the brain was affected. These can include physical, cognitive, and communication challenges that vary widely from person to person.

A stroke is also known as a *brain attack* or a *cerebrovascular accident (CVA)*. Strokes are not uncommon, and they can affect anyone at any age. Stroke is the fifth leading cause of death and the leading cause of adult disability in the United States, affecting nearly 800,000 people per year.

> *"I didn't understand stroke at all when I had mine. It would have been helpful if someone had drawn a picture of a brain and showed me how the left side of the brain controls the right side of the body. Videos or visuals would have been great since I had trouble understanding words. I've met many survivors who say they didn't understand much in the hospital and were scared. I hope this book gives you some of the information I needed when I first had a stroke."* — David

A Tip from Dr. Mike

As the saying goes, knowledge is power. The first step in this recovery journey is a better understanding of what has occurred. By learning *what* has happened to the brain during a stroke, you can then have a better idea of *how* you can best optimize recovery.

The Full Picture of Stroke

A stroke can cause problems with movement, vision, memory, sensation, communication, eating, or thinking skills. It can impair your ability to care for yourself in many ways. Since certain parts of the brain are specialized for specific functions, a stroke in one of these areas may cause particular challenges:

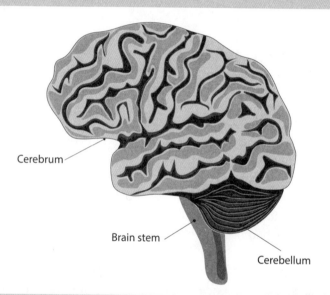

Cerebrum

Brain stem

Cerebellum

Left hemisphere of the cerebrum

- Right-sided weakness or sensory problems
- Language problems
- Impaired analytical skills

Right hemisphere of the cerebrum

- Left-sided weakness or sensory problems
- Visual-spatial problems
- Impulsivity or inappropriate behavior

Cerebellum
- Coordination and balance problems
- Dizziness

Brain stem
- Swallowing problems
- Vision issues
- Decreased alertness

2. What causes a stroke?

Dr. Roth: A stroke is any problem that results from blood vessel disease in the brain. There are several different kinds of problems that could happen with the blood vessels. The most common type of stroke—about 85 percent of all strokes—is an *ischemic* or *thrombotic* stroke. This is where there's a blockage, or *occlusion*, from a **clot** stuck in a blood vessel that goes up to the brain or in the brain itself. Any of the brain tissue that surrounds or is supplied by that particular blood vessel is then affected and becomes either injured or sometimes permanently damaged because of the lack of oxygen, blood supply, and nutrients.

The other type of stroke, which is less common—about 15 percent of all strokes—is a *hemorrhagic* stroke, or a **bleed** in the brain. That's when the blood actually leaves the blood vessel itself, goes into the brain tissue, and sort of pushes the brain tissue aside. In this case, the blood itself is actually pushing or damaging the neuron cells, so the nerves become affected. Any of the functions, behaviors, or activities that are controlled by that particular part of the brain are impacted and become abnormal.

Author's note: While fewer people have hemorrhagic strokes, they tend to be deadlier. People having a hemorrhagic stroke are more likely to have headaches, nausea, or seizures than those with ischemic strokes, but only a brain image can tell the difference for certain. Hemorrhagic strokes may be caused by high blood pressure or weakened blood vessels, known as aneurysms or *arteriovenous malformations* (AVMs).

3. Who is at risk for a stroke?

Dr. Roth: I put stroke risk factors into three broad categories. The first are risk factors that can be changed with **medication or medical treatment**, like surgical correction of blood vessel abnormalities, taking blood thinner medication, or taking an aspirin a day.

The second broad category is risk factors that can be changed with **lifestyle changes**. Things like controlling high blood pressure, diabetes, and cholesterol, or giving up a sedentary lifestyle, smoking, and alcohol.

The third are risk factors that cannot be changed. For example, **family history** increases the risk of having a stroke very slightly, and there are genetic conditions that can lead to a stroke (e.g., sickle-cell disease, Fabry disease, CADASIL). People like to talk about those things, but you can't do much about them.

Focus on the things that are changeable either through lifestyle or medicine.

"I had a stroke when I was just 10 years old because I have Moyamoya disease. It is a rare condition that prevents blood from flowing freely in the brain because the blood vessels get too small. There was nothing I could have done to prevent it. But you probably don't have a one-in-a-million brain disease like I have. There are many things you can do to prevent having a stroke. And for us survivors, there are many things we can do to prevent having another one." — David

A Tip from Dr. Mike

"I always tell my patients that feelings are information. And so it goes with anxiety, which has the power to either prevent or promote change in our lives. What is your anxiety telling you? Is it urging you to do something differently? Perhaps it's reminding you to see your specialist or get that physical you were supposed to have last year. Maybe it's begging you to eat better, drink less, start meditating, or exercise more. Or maybe it's telling you to talk to someone about your fears. When we allow anxiety to help us create positive change, we will probably have a little less anxiety in the future."

Dr. Chiu: There is a difference between the rate of stroke in men and the rate of stroke in women. The incidence of stroke is lower in women until around the age of menopause. So there's kind of a protective effect of being female, but once you get older that benefit seems to go away. In fact, because women tend to survive to older ages than men on average, there are actually significantly more women who end up suffering a stroke than men.

Another observation, in terms of the demographics of stroke, is that there is a "stroke belt" in the United States. That stroke belt encompasses the southeastern United States, where there is a dramatically higher rate of stroke—almost double that of the rest of the country. The reasons for that likely have to do with the known risk factors for stroke: dietary differences; the prevalence of high blood pressure, diabetes, and smoking; and some racial and ethnic differences in the rates of stroke as well.

African Americans are at higher risk for stroke, nearly twice that of Caucasians. Some conditions, like *intracranial atherosclerosis* (hardening of the arteries in the brain), are more prevalent among Hispanics and Asians.

There are also more young people having strokes now than ever before, and it has to do with the prevalence of stroke risk factors. As obesity becomes more rampant, diabetes becomes more prevalent, and drug abuse becomes more widespread, you're going to see an increase in the rates of stroke. Even children, infants, and newborns can have strokes. The good news is that there is greater brain plasticity to recover in younger people, though they have to deal with the impact of a stroke for many more years of their lives.

"I was a child when I had my stroke. That was good because my brain was more 'plastic' than an adult brain. Then again, my stroke was also far worse than most adult strokes. I recovered the way I did not just because of how plastic my brain was; it was also because of what I believed about the world. As a child, I thought people get sick and then they get better. I always believed I would get better. I had no idea that a stroke could cause a long-term disability. This belief became a self-fulfilling prophecy and kept hope alive. I hope you have the same sort of optimism I had. It may make a big difference in your recovery." — David

A Tip from Dr. Mike

"Core beliefs we have about ourselves and the world affect the way we think, feel, act, and recover. They have real, biological effects throughout our bodies and brains. If you believe 'Bad things always happen to me,' then you'll start to look for evidence of this. This can lead to hopelessness, which then leads to high levels of stress hormones. These stress hormones can create inflammation, which prevents your body and brain from healing. Even if you are struggling today, try to modify your core belief. For example, say, 'There are bad things happening right now, but I also know I still have good things in my life.' Then, look for evidence of this. By doing so, you'll have the power to change the way you think, feel, act, and heal. Create a core belief that inspires you. Remind yourself of this belief every day."

4. What are the chances that stroke survivors will have another stroke at some point in their lives?

Dr. Chiu: The risk of a stroke recurrence depends on what caused the stroke in the first place, and also which stroke risk factors that person had. There's no doubt about it—having a stroke puts any individual in a high-risk category for a stroke recurrence. So if you take a look at overall numbers, about 10 percent of all patients who have a stroke will suffer a second stroke in the first year. Now of course that risk can be modified greatly, depending on the treatment and preventive measures that one takes.

Dr. Roth: The risk of a second stroke after a first stroke depends on the type of stroke and the causes. For example, some people who have had a hemorrhagic stroke because of an abnormal blood vessel, like an aneurysm, will need surgery to have the aneurysm clipped or reduced. In that case, their risk of another stroke becomes much, much lower. But if it's not taken care of, obviously there's still a risk of a subsequent stroke.

Similarly, if a person who's had an ischemic stroke continues to have the same risk factors that caused the stroke in the first place—like high blood pressure, diabetes, smoking, or alcohol overuse—and none of those things are addressed, then that's a problem and the risk of recurrence goes up.

Author's note: At least a quarter of all stroke survivors will have another stroke in their lifetimes. You can dramatically lower your risk by knowing what caused your stroke and reducing your risk factors. However, in up to a third of strokes, the cause is unknown. These types of strokes are called *cryptogenic strokes*, and they can be frustrating and scary. Your doctor may be able to do further tests to determine the cause of your stroke and help you take steps to manage your risk factors to prevent a recurrent stroke.

5. What can someone do to prevent having a(nother) stroke?

Dr. Chiu: A few decades ago, it was thought that stroke was nearly untreatable. In the course of a few decades, we've gone from that to making stroke likely the most preventable of the catastrophic diseases. One of the bedrock principles of stroke prevention in patients who've had a stroke is to aggressively treat the stroke risk factors. We know a lot about the risk factors for stroke: high blood pressure (*hypertension*), high cholesterol, smoking, and obesity. So if we aggressively treat the modifiable risk factors, we see that can have a tremendous impact on the chances of having a recurrent stroke.

I'll give you a couple of examples of conditions that have tailored preventive measures.

Patients who have a condition called *atrial fibrillation*, a type of **irregular heartbeat** (or cardiac arrhythmia), are five times more likely to have a stroke than people their own age who don't have atrial fibrillation. So this is the most important of the *cardioembolic* causes of stroke—strokes that are caused by clots that form in the heart, break off, go up to the brain, and obstruct a blood vessel. Atrial fibrillation is a very important cause of stroke; it accounts for 15 percent or more of all ischemic strokes.

For patients who have atrial fibrillation, there is a highly effective treatment for stroke prevention called *anticoagulant therapy*, which helps prevent the blood from clotting. One of the major breakthroughs of the last five years has been the development of new oral **anticoagulant medications** that have, in many cases, overtaken the older Coumadin (warfarin) medications as the first-line choice for preventing stroke in patients with atrial fibrillation. These are drugs like Eliquis (apixaban), Pradaxa (dabigatran), and Xarelto (rivaroxaban), and they're highly effective. We're talking about drugs that by themselves can reduce the risk of stroke by 70 to 80 percent.

Another important cause of stroke is *carotid stenosis*, a **blockage of the carotid artery** in the neck, which is one of the major highways of blood flow to the brain. If you have a severe blockage in the carotid artery, it puts you at high risk for having a stroke. Often people with carotid stenosis will need *carotid revascularization,* a kind of surgery or procedure to open up the artery. We now have both the traditional surgical technique and a procedure called *carotid stenting,* which has been shown in recent years to be the equivalent of surgery in terms of the effectiveness of opening up the artery and preventing future strokes.

For patients who don't have atrial fibrillation or carotid stenosis, often they may benefit from taking medications like aspirin or clopidogrel (Plavix). These are **blood-thinning medicines,** and for patients with ischemic stroke they are often valuable in reducing the risk of a stroke recurrence.

Blood pressure control is absolutely critical. This is one of the things that can most accurately determine the likelihood of someone suffering another stroke. High blood pressure is almost definitely the most important, treatable risk factor for stroke, from a public health standpoint.

There are certain types of stroke that are directly a result of having chronic high blood pressure. For patients with *intracerebral hemorrhages* (the most common type of hemorrhagic stroke), high blood pressure is far and away the leading cause. High blood pressure is also the most important cause of a type of ischemic stroke called *lacunar stroke.*

There are a number of ways that you can control blood pressure after a stroke. You can do it by eating a healthy diet and reducing salt intake, exercising or being physically active, and, for a lot of people with high blood pressure, taking medication. We are recognizing more and more how important it is to keep the blood pressure optimally controlled—not just so-so, not high normal, but optimally controlled.

• • • • •

TAKEAWAY POINTS:

There are two types of strokes:

- The most common is an ischemic stroke, which is caused by a clot stuck in the blood supply of the brain; 85 percent of strokes are ischemic.
- The other type is a hemorrhagic stroke, which is caused by a bleed in the brain; 15 percent of strokes are hemorrhagic.

Anyone can have a stroke at any time in his or her life. However, some people have more risk factors for stroke. You can control many of these risk factors through lifestyle choices:

- Eating a low-sodium, heart-healthy diet
- Maintaining a healthy weight
- Being physically active
- Not smoking
- Limiting alcohol use

Talk to your doctor to see if you need:

- Anticoagulant medications for atrial fibrillation
- Surgery for carotid stenosis to clear the arteries to the brain
- Blood-thinning medication
- Blood pressure medication
- Cholesterol-lowering medication
- Diabetes management or better blood sugar control

Prevention is equally important before and after a stroke because many survivors remain at risk for another stroke. Controlling your blood pressure is the most important thing you can do.

CHAPTER 2

STROKE TREATMENT

Regardless of why it happened, a stroke must be treated—and fast. When you get to the hospital, you'll encounter specialized doctors and nurses who will diagnose and treat the stroke. We invited two of the best to join the conversation. Dr. Jan Hinkle is a clinical nurse specialist and president of the American Association of Neuroscience Nurses. Dr. Tom Carmichael is an acclaimed neurologist, neuroscientist, and the co-director of the UCLA Broad Stem Cell Research Center. Along with Dr. Chiu and Dr. Roth, they'll help explain what happens immediately after a stroke.

6. What should you do if you're having a stroke?

Dr. Hinkle: You can learn to recognize a stroke by using the acronym *FAST*. The *F* in *FAST* stands for face—sudden weakness on one side of your face. If you have sudden weakness in one of your arms—if you can't lift both arms—that's the *A*. If you have sudden problems with your speech, that's the *S*. The *T* is time. Time is brain—time to call 911. You shouldn't call your family doctor. Call an ambulance and get yourself to the nearest stroke center. The ambulance drivers generally will know where the closest stroke-certified hospital is that can give you the best treatment.

F = Face drooping
A = Arm weakness
S = Speech difficulty
T = Time to call for help

Author's note: Many people who are suffering a stroke think they just need to lie down for a few minutes, or that they'll feel better in the morning. Ignoring the symptoms of a stroke or delaying treatment can greatly reduce the ability of the doctors to provide brain-saving drugs and surgical procedures. This is what is meant by "time is brain."

"I had my stroke while on a family vacation. Looking back, there were a few early warning signs. Hours before my stroke, my uncle noticed me having trouble buttoning my shirt with my dominant right hand and using my left instead. I started feeling sick and took a nap in the hotel room with my mom. When I woke up, I couldn't talk. At first, my mom thought I was kidding. When I got to the emergency room, I went into seizures. Since I was only 10 when I had my stroke, my family and I weren't on the lookout for any warning signs, but you should be." — David

A Tip from Dr. Mike

"Most people who have a stroke are over 50, but the number of younger adults having strokes has spiked recently. While my brother's stroke was caused by a rare brain disease that couldn't have been reversed, most strokes in younger people are related to obesity, high blood pressure, diabetes, and smoking. No matter your age, be on the lookout for the warning signs of a stroke while addressing lifestyle choices that help prevent them. An ounce of prevention is worth a pound of cure."

7. Does it matter which hospital you go to?

Dr. Hinkle: Yes. There's been a movement in the last two decades to establish what's called *stroke systems of care*. These are integrated regional stroke facilities. They make sure there are agreements between the hospital and the emergency medical services (EMS) that are most commonly bringing people in via ambulance. They also make sure there's integration with the public and government agencies, so stroke survivors know where the resources are once they leave the hospital. The American Heart Association and the American Stroke Association now certify hospitals at three different levels in the stroke system of care: acute stroke–ready hospital, primary stroke center, and comprehensive stroke center.

About a third of hospitals in the United States are certified as being *primary stroke centers*, meaning that the emergency room has written protocols and everybody knows what to do when a stroke patient comes in. They have transfer agreements with other hospitals, they have a director of stroke care, and most important, they have the ability to give the right brain-saving drugs.

Author's note: Ask to be taken to a *stroke-certified* hospital if you have a choice. There are three levels of certification. An *acute stroke–ready hospital* (ASRH) has the ability to diagnose and treat strokes and can transfer you to a primary or comprehensive stroke center if needed. A *primary stroke center* (PSC) has more tools and specialists available, with designated beds and staff for stroke patients. There are over 1,000 PSCs in the United States. A *comprehensive stroke center* (CSC) has everything: dedicated intensive care for neurological patients, specialized neurosurgery, plus patient-centered stroke research. There are just over 100 CSCs in the United States today.

8. What will happen at the hospital?

Dr. Carmichael: Most commonly strokes are diagnosed with the clinical exam done by an emergency room physician or a neurologist, followed by some form of brain imaging—an MRI or CT scan.

There is a lot that can be done with early stroke therapies to limit the damage. So patients should expect a **fairly substantial and very quick workup** in the emergency department of a major hospital to understand the mechanism of the stroke, and, if there's salvageable brain tissue, what might be done to open the clotted artery and allow blood to flow back into that brain tissue.

9. What are the immediate treatments for a stroke?

Dr. Chiu: For ischemic strokes, there are things that we can do to potentially reverse the effects, or at the very least minimize the effects. But these are things that have to be done almost immediately. One treatment is what we call *mechanical clot retrieval*: going up into the artery of the brain with a catheter, snatching that clot, pulling it out, and restoring blood flow to that part of the brain.

Dr. Carmichael: There's one drug that's called *tPA* (tissue plasminogen activator), and it helps dissolve clots. You may have heard it called the **clot-busting drug**. It's been around since the late 1990s, and it is used for ischemic strokes. It has a very good effect the earlier you give it. The faster you can get a patient from the location of their stroke, say from the door of their home, to the hospital to receive the drug by IV, the better the outcome. Stroke doctors call this *door-to-needle time*. There's a very strong focus in most stroke units on quick transport of patients to the hospital and then administration of this drug. After about four-and-a-half hours, the risk of giving tPA outweighs the benefits.

10. When would a stroke survivor need surgery?

Dr. Carmichael: There are a couple of conditions related to a stroke itself when surgery is appropriate. In a certain percentage of patients with ischemic strokes, there will be swelling, or *edema*. That's called *malignant stroke*, when the stroke causes fluid from the rest of the brain to rush in. If the brain swells, the skull can't expand, so the brain will collapse in on itself. The surgeon goes in and removes a bit of the skull to allow the swollen brain to expand out, and not damage or push on adjacent healthy brain tissue.

Another indication for surgery is when the stroke is caused by a brain hemorrhage, which happens in 15 percent or so of strokes. Removing the hemorrhage by draining the blood or repairing the ruptured blood vessel can help reduce the symptoms on the adjacent brain tissue.

11. What is a ministroke, or TIA (transient ischemic attack)?

Dr. Chiu: The term *TIA*, versus the term *stroke*, is meant to denote that the symptoms, which are the same for the two, are transient, or temporary, with a TIA, so they resolve completely. Typically the effects will be observable for a few minutes to several hours, but the effects disappear within 24 hours.

It is very important that you **do not ignore** the symptoms of a TIA. The risk of a stroke after a TIA can be just as high, if not higher, as the risk of having a second stroke after a full-fledged stroke. This means that you need to seek medical attention immediately after a TIA, just as you would if you had actually suffered a full-fledged stroke. It also means that you now have an opportunity to take preventive measures so that you can avoid a full-fledged stroke, where the consequences can be permanent or long-term.

12. Are there any drugs available that can help the brain repair after a stroke?

Dr. Carmichael: Unfortunately, there is no real medical therapy that promotes brain repair at present. There are likely to be some in the next 5 to 10 years, but at the moment, there is no drug or pill that someone can take to enhance recovery in the brain.

However, there are a couple of roles for the selective serotonin reuptake inhibitors (SSRIs). These medicines, commonly known as Prozac (fluoxetine), Paxil (paroxetine), or Zoloft (sertraline), were originally developed for depression. One of their main and well-substantiated roles is in **treating poststroke depression**. Up to 30 percent of patients get clinically depressed after a stroke, and some of this may be from the stroke itself. Just like a stroke interrupts circuits that control movement, it can interfere with circuits that control emotion. So depression can be a real neurological side effect of a stroke, and people who are depressed after a stroke do not recover as well. So one clear benefit of using these drugs is to treat poststroke depression.

There was also one clinical study that suggested that Prozac, given in the first 90 days after a stroke, may enhance recovery of movement. This could have been because it enhanced the ability to engage in rehab and more fully participate by controlling depression, but there's also a signature in that data that it may indeed have enhanced recovery. So early after a stroke, in the first couple of weeks to months, there may also be a role for these SSRIs in enhancing recovery.

There have been small case reports or studies that suggest that boosting L-DOPA, using a Parkinson's disease drug such as Sinemet (carbidopa levodopa) or stimulants like Ritalin (methylphenidate) may help; but whenever attempts have been made to repeat those results or use larger case studies, they've never borne out.

The problem is that many physicians feel the need to do *something*, so patients end up on a lot of these drugs. One of the things we often do in neurorehab is take patients off the drugs to see how they do. If the drugs are helping, patients should deteriorate, in which case of course we put them back on the drugs. More often than not, they just sort of accumulate these drugs over time by seeing different physicians who want to help. The physicians prescribe the drugs, but all drugs do have side effects. So if there's no medical evidence to support them, it's usually not worth taking them because of the risk of side effects.

◇◇

A stroke survivor asks, "What other medical concerns do I now have to watch out for because I've had a stroke?"

Dr. Chiu: The obvious concerns, such as paralysis on one side of the body causing problems with motor function, or an impairment in speech or language, you know right away. Once the dust settles and someone who has been hospitalized for a stroke goes home, often it will become more evident if there are cognitive deficits.

However, another thing to watch out for is **dementia**. Many people think of Alzheimer's disease anytime the term *dementia* is used, but in fact strokes are the second leading cause of dementia after Alzheimer's. Cognitive problems that get worse over time instead of staying the same or improving may be related to *vascular dementia*.

Changes in mood, such as **depression**, can occur in as many as a third of patients after a stroke. This may become apparent only later, so it's important to watch for it.

Seizures can occur in about 10 percent of patients who have had a stroke. Sometimes seizures can be in the immediate aftermath of a stroke, and sometimes they can occur weeks, months, or even years after a stroke. Seizures happen because the scar tissue caused by a stroke results in the abnormal electrical firing of the brain cells.

Dr. Roth: People with strokes are actually at risk for a number of medical conditions, especially early after a stroke. For example **blood clots**, what we call DVT, or *deep vein thrombosis* (clots in the legs), and *pulmonary embolisms* (clots in the lungs), can be very serious complications and are fairly common. Up to 60 percent of people get those early on after a stroke, but the risk period goes away about a month or two following the stroke.

Likewise, having **infections** like pneumonia or a urinary tract infection can be fairly common. A lot of the complications come from *immobilization*, meaning not moving much, like **pressure ulcers or contractures** (stiffness or tightness of the limbs) as well as the blood clots. Those things are big problems of being sedentary and immobilized.

Dr. Hinkle: To help prevent blood clots in the legs, getting up and moving as much as possible as soon as possible is the key. If you are at high risk for DVT, the doctor will evaluate you for blood-thinning medications, such as low-dose Heparin, so the clots don't form as readily. If you see one leg looking larger than the other and it's red and swollen, call the doctor and don't massage the leg.

Bruising is going to happen more readily if you're on an anticoagulant medication. The biggest complication is the chance of a **gastrointestinal (GI) bleed**. So if you see blood in your stool, or unusual bleeding from anywhere, you want to call the doctor right away.

Talk to the team about what to expect from any new medications you're on.

◇◇◇

• • • • •

Takeaway Points:

Learn to identify a stroke by using the acronym *FAST*:

- **F**ace: Is the face drooping on one side?
- **A**rms: Can the person raise both arms?
- **S**peech: Is the speech clear and coherent?
- **T**ime: Now is the time to call 911!

Get to a stroke-certified hospital if possible, to get the best treatments. The neurologist will decide if the stroke patient needs the clot-busting drug, clot-removal, surgery, or other treatments.

After the immediate medical treatments, there are no drugs to speed recovery, although treating depression may be a good idea.

A ministroke (or TIA) requires the same medical attention as a full stroke.

After a stroke, be on the lookout for signs of these other complications that can result from inactivity, medications, or damage to the brain:

- Blood clots
- Bruising
- GI bleeds

- Pneumonia
- Urinary tract infections
- Pressure ulcers
- Contractures
- Depression
- Seizures
- Dementia

CHAPTER 3

WHAT TO EXPECT

A stroke happens in an instant, but recovery takes much longer. Every brain is different, and every stroke is unique, so it's hard to know exactly what your recovery will look like. Some people make a full and rapid recovery, while others regain some abilities more slowly. However, there are some general trends in stroke recovery that can help you know what to expect and how to maximize your improvement. Dr. Carmichael and Dr. Roth share their expertise from working with stroke survivors in their medical practices and research.

13. What are the stages of stroke recovery?

Dr. Carmichael: There are stages of stroke recovery that are fairly well recognized, although there's still some debate about their precise boundaries. Early on there's the **hyperacute stage**. This means the stroke and tissue damage are evolving within minutes, so decisions must be made very fast in terms of opening the blood clot or other therapeutic options, often by the stroke neurologist.

The **acute stage** is within the few days following the stroke. It still occurs within the stroke unit in the hospital, but there are no longer medical therapies directed at the vessel that was blocked. The clot opens for everyone within the first three days—no matter whether you get a drug or a stent or anything. Now is when we focus on stabilizing the patient, understanding why the stroke occurred, and getting them ready for the next stage of recovery.

The next stage is the **subacute stage**. This happens after the first five or six days and lasts about three to six months. It's when most of the recovery occurs. Fortunately, this recovery happens almost no matter what you do—it's *spontaneous recovery.* So it doesn't matter if a patient is in a rehab unit, at home with therapy, or in a skilled nursing facility—all patients get progressively better during this phase.

Then after this three- to six-month subacute phase, we enter the **chronic stage** of stroke recovery. In the chronic stage, **recovery is still possible**, though it may be slower and more *task specific.* Whereas in the subacute period recovery is more general and occurs across walking, speaking, and using the arm, in the chronic phase, it's really more about improving on one task at a time, and it requires more effort.

Recovery with a chronic stroke is usually in one area that the patient is really motivated to work on. Patients may say, "My walking is impaired, and that's the thing I really want to improve." So they would then focus on rehabilitative therapies toward walking. Or they may say, "It's my reach and my grasp—that's really what I want to focus on." So they would focus on that with a therapist or exercises. It takes more work and more time, but they can make progress.

14. How long will it take to recover?

Dr. Roth: Recovery differs in every single patient. There are some people who have a more or less consistent upward trend in their abilities, and there are some people for whom it happens in fits and starts, making progress then leveling off, then making progress again. Sometimes people don't improve a lot early on, and then they start to improve a whole lot later. So it really varies.

One thing that's important to keep in mind is that there are two broad categories of recovery for people who have had a stroke. It can be the recovery of the *impairments,* such as improved arm strength, improved leg strength, or improved language and communication, or it can be the recovery of *function*—day-to-day tasks such as being able to walk, get dressed, or take care of oneself, even if the arm or leg is weak or the language is not fully recovered.

The old textbooks often say that recovery stops or slows after a certain point—anywhere from three to six months is often quoted—but every one of us who works in rehabilitation sees patients continue to improve long after that. Sometimes it is actually the physical recovery (improvement of the impairment), but more often it's actually improvement in the ability to be independent, the ability to do some of the day-to-day activities on their own (improvement of function).

Dr. Carmichael: It's somewhat of a misperception that there's a limit to recovery at a certain time, and unfortunately some doctors perpetuate this. It's distressing when I have patients come to me and say, "Well, the doctor told me that I was never going to move the arm again," and I realize that the doctor was an emergency room physician who by definition sees emergencies and doesn't see things over time. Perhaps a neurologist who doesn't have a lot of experience in chronic-stroke recovery will make some hasty statement about a limit or a ceiling on recovery. If patients can connect with doctors who see recovery over time, who know the emerging research findings, then they will be more likely to get a better idea of how far they can expect to go.

As for making a full recovery, it depends on the person's age and the type of stroke. After a mild stroke, many patients will achieve full recovery. If a stroke is substantial but the patient is very young, the person may achieve full recovery. For the bulk of stroke patients, those who are adults and have medium-size strokes, full recovery is usually not seen, but *meaningful recovery* and regaining lost activities are reasonable goals and are possible.

15. What factors impact stroke recovery?

Dr. Carmichael: A number of factors have really powerful interactions with stroke recovery. One is **age**—the younger the brain is, the more it recovers. The older one is, the more age has a negative effect on recovery. A second factor is **where in the brain** the stroke occurred. If a stroke wipes out some of the pathways from the brain down to the spinal cord, recovery is substantially reduced. **Stroke size** has an important interaction, although not as much as you might think. Whether the critical parts of the brain are hit by a stroke is more important, but in general, bigger strokes are associated with less recovery. Then there are **medical conditions**, such as poorly controlled diabetes, that can impact recovery.

The overall **motivation** and **physical activity** levels of patients frequently impact recovery as well. I often see patients go home and become increasingly less active. It's such a bummer to see that because stroke patients are uniquely sensitive to inactivity, and they lose their recovered functions quite quickly if they don't use them. So stroke is actually now seen as a chronically progressive illness rather than what it should be, which is an acute event that we then recover from slowly. Instead, a lot of stroke patients go home, achieve such little activity that they lose the recovery they had initially gained in rehab, and end up, five years down the road, in worse shape than they were in three months after the stroke. That's largely due to inactivity. It really is a case of **use it or lose it**.

It can be a vicious cycle. It's obviously harder to do the physical things you used to do; yet it becomes more important than ever to do them. A really good chronic-stroke medical team can work with patients to try to identify activities that are pleasurable so that the motivation remains high, but that provide a graduated increase in challenge so that patients can continue to progress in their recoveries.

Dr. Roth: Clearly a big factor affecting stroke recovery is **the stroke itself**: the size, the location, the type of injury to the brain, how much inflammation there is, and the blood supply to the brain. There are other physical factors as well, such as medical stability, endurance, and the ability to participate in therapy.

I tell all my patients and family members that determination is half of the battle. **Motivation and determination** mean a great deal. They don't account for everything, but they do mean a lot. So much of the recovery process after a stroke has to do with what an individual does him- or herself, how hard he or she works, how much effort he or she puts into it.

We practice what we call a *bio-psycho-social model of care* in rehabilitation. Certainly the biological factors are important, but those factors do not drive the entire process. A big part of recovery is what the individual puts into it, how he or she feels about it, and how much support there is—socially, spiritually, and psychologically. Having a supportive family and a supportive environment along with community resources can be extremely valuable.

"It is important for patients to stay positive. No one can predict your recovery. One doctor told my mom I would not recover much and suggested I be placed in a nursing home. Luckily, she did not listen to him. I improved slowly but steadily over the years. I'm not in a nursing home. Hopefully you will surprise people with your recovery." — David

A Tip from Dr. Mike

"Every day, find three simple and specific things you are grateful for. If you took one extra step in physical therapy today, take a moment to appreciate your progress. If they're serving your favorite food for lunch today, take a moment to give thanks. This simple practice can help you to stay positive throughout the recovery journey. Maintaining a positive outlook can have a profound effect."

16. What is neuroplasticity, and how does it impact stroke recovery?

Dr. Carmichael: *Neuroplasticity* is the way the circuits in the brain can change and take new shapes. We take advantage of this **amazing ability of our brains to change** in order to promote greater recovery of function after a stroke. We all use neuroplasticity all the time when we're forming new memories or learning new things. In stroke patients, the brain tissue that survived can take on some of the function of the tissue that was lost.

When we image the brains of people recovering from a stroke, we see that the brains are active but in inefficient ways. Lots of areas are firing, but there aren't clear patterns or networks. Then, as patients learn how to recover through practice and task-specific activities, we see these networks start to become more strongly activated together into a *recovery network*. So the brain uses the practice and the extra effort patients put in to essentially teach a new network of neurons to perform the function that was lost, whether it's speech or movement or sensation. However, the brain really hates to form this alternative network. That's why it goes away so fast when you're inactive. You can get it back again, but it takes constant reinforcement to keep a brain recovery network active and connected.

17. What are some things stroke survivors can do to maximize this neuroplasticity?

Dr. Carmichael: There are promising drugs that may become available in the next 7 to 10 years to enhance plasticity and promote recovery. But for now, the main thing is to use the affected function regularly, every day. Even though it's a struggle, each day **devote time and effort** to using the function that doesn't work.

10 Principles of Neuroplasticity

The best stroke therapies exploit how neuroplasticity works by using **repetitive, positive experiences** to forge and strengthen pathways in the brain. Here are the 10 principles of experience-dependent neuroplasticity:

1. Use it or lose it: The skills you don't practice often get weaker.
2. Use it and improve it: The skills you practice get better.

3. Specificity: You must skillfully practice the exact tasks you want to improve.

4. Repetition matters: You must do a task over and over again once you've got it right to actually change the brain.

5. Intensity matters: More repetitions in a shorter time are necessary for creating new connections.

6. Time matters: Neuroplasticity is a process rather than a single event, with windows of opportunity opening for different skills at different times. In rehabilitation, starting earlier is usually better than starting later.

7. Salience matters: To change the brain, the skill you're practicing must have some meaning, relevance, or importance to you.

8. Age matters: Younger brains tend to change faster than older brains, but improvement is possible at any age.

9. Transference: Practicing one skill can result in improvement of a related skill.

10. Interference: Learning an easier way of doing something (i.e., a bad habit or compensation) may make it harder to learn the proper way.

Whether you're learning a new skill or relearning a lost one, it's clear you must practice the thing you want to get better. There are no quick fixes.

"I started with no movement on the right side, and progress was slow. I'm now able to walk and run without a leg brace. I still can't use my right hand to pick up something or write, but I can use it to hold a napkin while eating. Therapy has also helped me to gain more mobility in my right shoulder and upper

arm. Therapy is hard, and sometimes I hate it. But you have to remind yourself that there is no gain without pain. You have to work through it. Focus on how worth it the end result will be."
— *David*

A Tip from Dr. Mike

"Permanence is what I refer to as a *pitfall thought pattern*. When we're feeling frustrated or sad, mood-congruent recall in the brain lights up all the memories with the same emotional charge. On sad days, all the sad memories in your brain light up, creating the illusion that you've always been sad, and thus, it feels like you always will be sad. The illusion of permanence is created. Talk back to this feeling by remembering another difficult time in your life that felt like it would never end—but did. This gives the logical part of you some evidence that can talk to the emotional part of you. It's saying, 'We've gotten through other tough times. We'll get through this too. Things will get better.'"

18. What can family members do after a stroke?

Dr. Carmichael: It is a very tense time. Emotions are running high. There are usually several family members involved with varying degrees of understanding. Things are moving fast, so it can lead to misunderstanding, uncertainty, and a lot of anxiety. One thing that can help is for the family to **establish a structured communication tree**, with one person taking the lead. Then the medical professionals can communicate well and often with that one person, rather than at different times with a lot of people who get a slightly different story each time. Clear communication with one or two designated family members helps to maximize the information the family gets and can act on and then allows the physicians to move quickly through an emergency situation.

Dr. Roth: We rely on the family members to be an important part of the team. Family members can provide a great deal of **emotional support**. Sometimes it's just by being there, sometimes it's by listening, and sometimes it's by being the ones to encourage, push, force, or bribe—whatever it takes to motivate the individual.

Sometimes family members provide a lot of the **physical help**. We almost always teach families how to do the exercises, how to help transfer a patient in and out of bed, how to push a wheelchair, how to help a patient go to the bathroom; so the training of caregivers or family members becomes a key element in the process.

Our role is to provide education and emotional support to the family as well as the patient so the family can do everything they can to maximize the rehabilitation of the individual with the stroke. Stroke really does happen to the family, not just the individual. We need the patient, family, and medical professionals to **work as a team** toward common goals to maximize recovery.

Your Recovery Team

We know that doctors and nurses will be part of the medical team at the hospital, but there are many other people involved—more than you might think. We've already met three of the professionals you'll encounter right away:

- Neurologist: a doctor who understands the brain and helps diagnose a stroke and determines the best treatment

- Physiatrist: a doctor who specializes in rehabilitation for physically disabling conditions like stroke, and focuses most heavily on improving function in daily life

- Nurse: a health-care worker who is there 24/7 to evaluate, treat, educate, assist, and provide care for patients in the hospital after a stroke

You'll meet so many other health-care professionals in the hospital too, and each one plays a special role requiring specialized knowledge and skills. You may encounter:

- Physical therapists: there to help you regain your physical strength and mobility

- Occupational therapists: there to help you reengage in your activities of daily living

- Speech-language pathologists: there to help you with communication and swallowing

- Recreational therapists: there to address your needs and maximize your strengths through recreation

- Music therapists: there to maximize your functioning through the power of music

- Social workers: there to support you and connect you with resources you'll need in your community

- Psychotherapists: there to help you adjust to life after a stroke or measure your cognitive skills

- Dieticians: there to ensure you're getting a healthy diet with the nutrition you need to heal

- Pharmacists: there to manage your medications and watch out for interactions and side effects

- And many others

In the next part, we'll look at how these professionals can help you as you recover. But remember, the most important members of your stroke recovery team are **you and your family**. It's *your* stroke, *your* life, and *your* recovery.

• • • • •

Takeaway Points:

Every stroke is different, but you can continue to recover function well beyond the first few months with task-specific goals and lots of effort. You can't control the size or location of your stroke or your age, but you can control your motivation, determination, and activity to have a better recovery.

Neuroplasticity is on your side. Use it or lose it; use it and improve it. Recovery is hard work that takes lots of repetition to change the brain. Families should establish a point person who will take the lead on all communication with the medical team and then distribute that information to the rest of the family. Families can also provide emotional support and physical help.

PART II:

YOUR THERAPY

CHAPTER 4

RECOVERING YOUR MOBILITY

Usually, the most noticeable effect of a stroke is paralysis or weakness on one side of the body. This is called *hemiparesis* (half-weak) or *hemiplegia* (half-paralyzed), and it can make it difficult to walk or even stand up. The weak or paralyzed side of the body is called the *affected* side. (Remember, one side of your brain controls the opposite side of your body. So if the medical team calls your stroke a "right CVA," they mean it's a cerebrovascular accident in the right hemisphere of your brain, even though you'll notice it on the left side of your body.) Building up strength and control of your body is a top priority after a stroke. Dr. Michelle Ploughman, a neurological physical therapist and top neurorehabilitation researcher, shares her expertise on how you can maximize your physical recovery and mobility.

19. What are the common physical effects of a stroke?

Dr. Ploughman: Strokes are quite variable from person to person. It depends on what side of the brain and which specific areas are affected. Most commonly, we see an **inability to move** the limbs on the affected side, due to *paralysis*.

Sometimes people experience *spasticity*, which means the muscles have too much activation. This is caused by the brain not being in full control of the muscles. It can be painful, with **spasms and tight muscles.**

Along with weakness and paralysis, there can be *sensory loss*. You feel **numbness and tingling** in your hands or feet, and you don't have a good sense of where your arm or leg is in space.

20. How can physical therapy help stroke survivors?

Dr. Ploughman: After a stroke, the brain goes through a period of inflammation and then repair. We call this *spontaneous recovery*. As inflammation within the brain subsides, movement on the affected side begins to emerge. This spontaneous recovery usually happens first in the midline of the body—so in the trunk and the hips first—and then it spreads to joints farther out from the center, such as the knee or elbow.

Physical therapists have two main roles. First, they want to **encourage more spontaneous recovery**, so they help the person with a stroke use the affected side as normally as possible. You might think that would be fairly simple, but it's not. Because humans are optimizers, in order to function in our world successfully, we use the abilities we have. So after a stroke, we tend to use our stronger side more and our affected side less. Physical therapists work hard to promote *symmetry* (equal ability on both sides) and to get the person with the stroke to use the affected side as the spontaneous recovery happens.

The second role of the physical therapist is to **strengthen the weak muscles**. Perhaps they are improving and recovering, but they're weak, so they need to be strengthened. The muscles need to learn when to turn on and off at the right time for agility and coordination. **Balance** has to be retrained, as well as the ability to move around and do functional tasks like rolling over in bed, standing from a seated position, walking, and climbing stairs. All those *motor programs* stored in our heads are lost because of a stroke, and we need to relearn them.

Author's note: In addition to therapy, doctors may be able to help with spasticity by giving injections of Botox. The same medicine used to remove wrinkles on your face can be used to relax tight muscles without the drowsiness caused by oral muscle relaxers. Botox can be injected directly into the tight muscles that are causing you the most pain.

21. How can exercise help with stroke recovery?

Dr. Ploughman: Exercise is really the foundation of stroke recovery. It's absolutely essential. It's important to know the different types of exercise, since not all exercises are created equal. In terms of neurorehabilitation, we think about three main types of exercise.

One is **intensive task practice**. Take an everyday task you want to focus on—for example, reaching for a pen or a cup. You break that task down into the components of the movement, and then practice the components thousands of times. Then you put the movement back together.

Another type of exercise is **strengthening** a weak muscle. You challenge the muscle so that it gains the power to hold and support the body.

The third type is **aerobic training**. What we know is that people with strokes have reduced functional capacity, so they feel tired doing everyday tasks. You need to do aerobic training to build your functional capacity so you can walk for long distances, for example, like getting across a large parking lot.

If you have a stroke, your physical capacity is lessened and you're not able to do as much, so your aerobic fitness goes down. Then, when you try to do a task, you feel more fatigued so you do less, and it becomes a vicious cycle. What you need to do is focus more on aerobic fitness. It will hopefully increase your capacity to do activities and decrease your fatigue so you'll be able to do more.

◇◇

A stroke survivor says, "I'm in a wheelchair. How can I exercise?"

Dr. Ploughman: Exercising from a wheelchair is certainly a challenge. Because your trunk is supported by the wheelchair, you're not free to move as easily as if you were sitting in a kitchen chair. If you are in a wheelchair, you can remove or flip aside the footrests to try to propel the chair forward and backward with your feet. This can help improve the coordination and movement of your legs. Done on a flat surface, it can help your timing and coordination, which is important for walking.

If you try the same activity on a slope, it will improve the power of your leg muscles and also bring in your abdominal and back muscles. However, it would be better to transfer to a regular chair or onto a piece of exercise equipment than stay in the wheelchair, if that's possible for you.

Author's note: There are many ways to perform aerobic training without walking, running, or playing sports—the things we typically think of as ways to get the heart rate up. You can use an arm or leg *ergometer* (pedaler), ride a stationary bike, swim or walk in a pool, or do chair aerobics (there are classes and videos for this). As you regain your strength and mobility, you can add activities like climbing stairs, rowing, dancing, or cycling. A recumbent tricycle is popular with stroke survivors who want to get exercise outdoors.

◇◇◇◇◇◇◇◇◇◇◇◇◇◇◇◇◇◇◇◇◇◇◇◇◇◇◇◇◇◇◇◇◇◇◇◇◇◇

22. What can stroke survivors do at home to improve their walking?

Dr. Ploughman: What research shows us is that the best way to improve walking is to walk. The theory is that it is *task-specific training*—the brain has motor programs that have already been formed for this task. So to access and train those programs, you have to **train specifically for what you want to do**. For example, studies have shown that practicing walking over ground is better than walking on a treadmill. Because ground is the real world, your body and brain remember how to do it.

You need to find ways that you can practice walking at home that are **safe**. Think about a short, safe space that you can walk along, either by holding on to another person, holding on to your kitchen counter, or using your cane and your kitchen counter. First you practice walking a small distance that you know is safe, a distance where your risk of falling is very, very low. If you're really unsteady, you might think turning around is a tricky movement to do. In this case, practice walking back and forth without turning around: walk backward five or six steps, then ahead five or six steps.

As you feel stronger and more confident, you're going to add to your distance by walking more laps back and forth. Then you will gradually begin to loosen your hold on the counter or a helper's hand, or switch from a rail to a cane, and from a cane to no cane. But be patient and build on your walking skills over time. It could take months or even years to reach your goals.

◇◇◇

A stroke survivor says, "The doctor said I'll probably never walk again. Is that true?"

Dr. Ploughman: I don't think anyone can tell a person that he or she won't walk again. **There is always hope** that you can. I'm a physical therapist as well as a neuroscientist, so I would ask, "Why can't you walk?" I would have to assess the person with the stroke to know. Is it because there's spasticity in the limbs that prevent the muscles from moving properly? Is it because the person has *contractures*, or tightness in the joints, and the joints won't flex and move? Is it because the person has fatigue and low aerobic capacity so he or she can't tolerate the exercise? Or is it poor balance? You have to find out the reasons why and then focus on improving those pieces to get back to walking.

◇◇◇

23. How does a person know when he or she is ready for a new walker or cane?

Dr. Ploughman: One way to know is that you feel it. As you're working on your walking, you'll start to feel a sense of confidence. Your confidence is saying, "I think I can actually stand here with one-finger support," or "I don't need this white-knuckle death grip on a cane." Once you get the sense that you're not putting much weight through your hand or that your hands are really doing very little, then you can start to reduce your *base of support.*

Think about your walker and cane as a base of support. A big walker with four wheels or four legs has a huge base of support—support that you need if your legs don't work properly and you have to use your hands to support yourself. If you feel like you're not using that base of support, you can probably move to a cane that has four points on it. Maybe that's enough—it's only a third of the size of the walker. Then if you feel that you're solid on the four legs of that cane, that you're not really using the cane that much, you can go with just a single-point cane.

24. What is foot drop? What can be done about it?

Dr. Ploughman: When you hear the term *foot drop*, it sounds pretty straightforward: the foot just drops. Actually, foot drop is complicated because it can be caused by a lot of different problems. There are two stages to walking: first you put weight on your leg, and then you swing your other leg through. With foot drop, the problem is that as you swing the affected leg through, your foot drags along the ground. This could be caused by **weakness** in the muscles in your shin that pull your foot up to clear the floor. It could be **tightness** in your calf muscles—an overactivation of spastic muscles in the calf can make the foot point downward and cause the toes to drag. Or it could be that the **hip, knee, and trunk** are not lifting the leg high enough.

Treatment for foot drop depends on what the problem is. There are some new devices on the market that stimulate the muscles on the front of the leg to lift the foot. So if the problem is that your foot doesn't lift, you can use muscle stimulation to help lift the foot. Sometimes the answer is a splint. You can place a splint inside your shoe to keep the foot up so that it doesn't drop down. This is called an *ankle-foot orthosis*, or AFO. But there is a down side to using an AFO. When you're trying to promote recovery in your ankle, having a splint to stop the ankle from moving isn't good. It's much better to practice and see if you can get that movement back without a splint.

If you're experiencing foot drop, you can meet with your physical therapist to determine which of the causes are responsible for the foot drop and then determine an appropriate treatment.

◇◇

A stroke survivor says, "I have the feeling of pins and needles in my leg all the time. What can I do about it?"

Dr. Ploughman: Many people with strokes have this feeling of buzzing through the limb, as though the leg is asleep and just waking up. It's often because the stroke has affected the sensory areas in the surface of the brain, or deep within the brain, and it can be really annoying.

There are two approaches for treatment. One is medication, so talk to your doctor about that. The other is a physical and sensory approach. The *gate theory of pain* proposes that your body can process only so much sensory information at one time. So if you touch, squeeze, or apply heat or cold to the limb, it can trick the sensory system into reducing the pins-and-needles feeling and starting to feel the other sensations.

Try to use your leg as much as possible. The brain is trying to rewire, and these pins and needles are sometimes caused by excessive plasticity—connections being made that are not helpful to you. So you want to give the leg as many normal sensations as you can: pressure, touch, standing, putting your weight through it, cold, heat—all those different sensations.

◇◇

25. How can stroke survivors maximize their physical recovery?

Dr. Ploughman: What we know about stroke recovery is that intensity matters. You have to practice certain movements thousands of times to regain and improve them. It won't happen by sitting down and doing nothing. You really have to map out that time to do it yourself, or get the help of a therapist, and engage all your family members.

Those people who come by and say, "Can I give you a hand? Is there anything I can do for you?"—tell them "Yes!" Ask them to do activities with you so you can get the practice in. You have to take advantage of the family and friends who are all around you, offering to help. They often want to help, but they don't know how, so they bake cookies or send flowers. Instead, you can **put them to work helping with therapy** through some very concrete tasks. If someone could just stand by you while you do your arm or leg exercises, that would be a tremendous help.

We know that the formal therapy you need is not always available. Even when it is, you maybe get five hours of therapy a week. But there are at least 12 waking hours in every day. *What are you doing for the rest of that time to promote recovery?*

In your first six months poststroke, your brain reverts back to a developmental stage. A lot of the proteins required for plasticity are strongly present in the brain in those first six months, so that's when you want to capitalize on everything around you. Have your therapists map out activities for you to do. Beyond the hour or so you spend with them a couple of times a week, take more hours—up to six a day broken up into periods—and **work hard on your rehab** during that six months when plasticity is at its highest.

26. What can be done to prevent falls in stroke survivors?

Dr. Ploughman: Falls are very common in stroke survivors and can be devastating because they can cause further injury. About 30 percent of people who are discharged from the hospital after a stroke will have a fall. Falls usually happen in the home. The riskiest time is in those first few weeks after discharge for people who use a walking aid or need assistance when walking. Falls are also more common in people who have depression.

Prevention is always better than cure. To prevent falls, especially in those first few weeks, you must make sure you have the assistance you need when you're moving. Falls usually happen when you let your mind drift for a moment, when you're in an unfamiliar environment, or when you're rushing. **Plan out your movement**—look at your space, picture your movements in your mind, and make sure you have enough help and the right footwear and equipment.

Remove all the things that cause clutter in your home. Remove throw rugs, relocate any wires or cords in your walking path, and move side tables or lamps that may get in your way. Bathrooms are a common place for falls because there's limited space and there are multiple obstacles around you. Install a rail or two in long hallways, and put grab bars in bathrooms to help.

• • • • •

Takeaway Points:

A stroke can leave you with a number of physical problems that can be helped by physical therapy:

- Paralysis or weakness
- Spasticity or tightness
- Sensory loss
- Decreased aerobic capacity
- Decreased balance

There are three types of exercise that are important to do:

1. Intensive task practice
2. Muscle strengthening
3. Aerobic activity

The best way to improve walking is by walking. Find a safe place to practice taking a few steps; then build on that. As you build strength, you can reduce how much support you need from walkers and canes. Talk to your doctor and physical therapist if you're experiencing the common poststroke problem of tingling in the limbs or foot drop. Ask family and friends to help you with your exercises. You need all the practice you can get for a better recovery.

Prevent falls before they happen by removing barriers and clutter, installing rails and safety equipment, and planning your movement before you start.

CHAPTER 5

RECOVERING YOUR ARM AND HAND

While losing your mobility can be devastating, it can be equally frustrating, if not more so, to lose the use of your arm and hand too. Our daily lives seem to require two hands to do just about everything—dressing, washing, cooking, working. We talked with three top occupational therapists and researchers to bring you answers about recovering the use of your affected *upper extremity* (arm and hand). Dr. Mary Ellen Stoykov is a researcher in the area of poststroke upper-limb hemiparesis and a professor at Rush University in Chicago. Dr. Glen Gillen is a professor at Columbia University who literally wrote the book on stroke rehabilitation—two textbooks and countless other publications. And Dr. Stephen Page leads the B.R.A.I.N. Lab as a professor at The Ohio State University and co-developed the stroke-specialist certification program for rehabilitation therapists.

27. Why is it that the paralyzed arm and hand seem the slowest to recover?

Dr. Stoykov: There are some pretty good reasons for that. One is the location of the stroke. The *middle cerebral artery* (MCA) is most commonly affected by stroke, and that artery covers a huge territory in the brain, which includes the area that controls the hand and the arm. We have more cortex area in the brain for controlling the hand and the arm than we have for controlling the leg. The reason is that our hand and arm movement is very sophisticated. It's harder to rehabilitate very complicated movement where lots of joints are involved than it is to rehabilitate walking, which is mostly hip flexion and knee extension. Walking is complicated, but arm movement is much more complicated.

An everyday action such as picking up an empty cup requires a lot of movements. First it requires movement in the shoulder; then the elbow has to straighten. Next, the forearm has to be placed at the exact angle in order for the hand to position itself and bring the fingers around the cup in the right shape and size. It's not as simple as it might seem.

28. What can stroke survivors do to get their hands working again?

Dr. Stoykov: One approach I advocate is **sensory feedback** into the hand. If you don't have movement, I would flood that hand with sensory feedback: rubbing a towel on it, applying vibrations, putting it in uncooked rice. We have connections in the brain that run between the sensory and motor cortices. They're very intricate connections, and sometimes when we massage or stimulate the sensory system, all of a sudden we see movement.

We take advantage of the two-way street between the brain and the hand. Even if the hand is not ready to move when the brain signals it to, you can put sensation in that hand so that it sends a message back to the brain to strengthen neural connections.

An occupational therapist can help you figure out things you can do in your life to get your arm moving. If there's no movement, or if the task is unsafe, there may also be one-handed techniques you can learn. But I'm not a fan of starting with those right away. It's use it or lose it, so you really want to try to **use your hand** to get that part of the brain that's affected by the stroke to work as much as possible.

The occupational therapist can help you learn to use that hand, even if only to use it as a stabilizer. For instance, you can use the affected hand to hold a jar while you open it with the other hand. Or you can use it to stabilize a piece of paper when writing. You can even just place your hand on a faucet and turn your arm to turn on the water, or you can put your hand on a doorknob and open and close it with your arm. Once you take the weight off the arm, the arm can move more easily than it would if it were moving against gravity.

Even if you don't have hand movement, **keep your arm moving** to decrease pain. Keeping a limb still is going to cause a pain syndrome. Continue any stretches or exercises you were given, and keep up activity in your life—you may be surprised what helps or happens as you're living your life. I've seen people who got memberships to a fitness center near where I work and came back in later with greatly improved arm movement. Well, it's because they were using some of the weight machines, and the more you use the hand and arm, the more it sends messages to the brain, and the more recovery happens.

29. Is there a time frame for regaining use of the upper extremity?

Dr. Stoykov: The first year is when you have the most chance of getting the movement back, but that does not mean that the movement is not going to come back after the first year. I've seen people in our research studies who get movement back after five years. The key is to try to use your arm as much as possible. But if you've reached a plateau and you want to move on with your life (i.e., stop going to therapy or being in research studies), then do that. If you see a change or start to get some movement back, then ask your doctor to give you another referral for occupational therapy based on the new movement that you have.

As with all other parts of stroke recovery, age, stroke location, and severity have an impact on upper extremity recovery too. Younger people tend to do better than elderly stroke survivors. But I would never say that you're never going to get movement back, because the brain is just too tricky. You may get some movements, but not a fully functional hand. Every little bit helps.

30. What is learned nonuse?

Dr. Gillen: The term *learned nonuse* is usually used to refer to people who have motor deficits on one side of the body. They can't use their bodies the same way they used to, so over time, they stop trying.

Let me give you an example of how it occurs. Let's say you have a stroke on the left side of your brain, so now your dominant right arm and leg have substantial weakness. The first time you start moving your body after the stroke, you don't realize what the deficits are. If you wake up the next morning after your stroke and breakfast is served, you're going to try to use your limbs the way you have previously. You might try to pick up your orange juice with your right hand, but because of the weakness, you might knock it over or spill it on yourself. So you start to get negative reinforcement for trying to use your limb.

Then it might be time to use the toilet, and you're going to try to stand up with both legs like you always have, but now your right leg might buckle on you. Again, you get negative reinforcement. All the therapists and nurses are telling you to try to use your right side, but when you try to use your right side to feed yourself, it takes 45 minutes and you're covered in food and drink and you're not comfortable. It makes sense then that you will start to use your nondominant, functioning left side. Because if you use your left side to eat breakfast, you're going to be able to eat in a reasonable amount of time, you're not going to be spilling things on yourself, you're not going to be knocking things over, and you're going to get positive reinforcement for using the nonaffected side. What happens, in fact, is that you learn not to use the side that's affected by the stroke. It's very difficult to remediate learned nonuse, but the technique we use is called *constraint-induced movement therapy* (CIMT).

31. What is constraint-induced movement therapy and who is a good candidate?

Dr. Page: Constraint-induced movement therapy is a protocol that helps to overcome learned nonuse with forced use. First, the therapist identifies tasks that are important to the patient and breaks them down. Then, as the patient becomes more proficient at performing the pieces of those tasks with the affected limb, the patient puts the pieces together. The second part of the program is to *constrain* the less affected arm, thus **forcing more use of the affected arm**. This is done by putting a padded mitt or glove on the good hand or by putting the good arm in a sling. Then the stroke survivor practices everyday tasks with only the affected hand or arm.

It's been proven that when you combine these pieces—have people practice iteratively using the arm, force use of the arm when they're home, and provide strategies to encourage them to use the arm at home (like keeping an exercise log)—it significantly improves arm function.

Traditionally, CIMT is administered very intensively over a two-week period, requiring people to go to therapy for six hours a day. There are a couple of problems with this: it's hard for patients to comply with the six-hour-a-day regimen, and it's hard to get reimbursed by insurance. Fortunately, we can modify the therapy and get similar results. We can do the therapy in half-hour segments three to four times a week with lots of home practice over a 10-week period and get the same results as with the intensive program. This is called *modified constraint-induced movement therapy* (mCIMT).

You shouldn't just do this on your own at home. The therapist guidance is important; therapists can assign the specific home exercises, check in on the progress of those exercises, modify them if they're too easy or too tough, and move forward from there. Ask your occupational therapist about whether it's right for you.

CIMT does not work for every stroke survivor. The program takes only people who have a little bit of active movement in the wrist and fingers—specifically what's called *extension*—and only about 25 percent of stroke survivors get that back. I get calls from people all the time who say, "I want to do constraint-induced therapy," because it's well publicized, but in fact it works only on the proportion of patients who have that active movement. It's a wonderful therapy, but as with any other area of medicine, we want to apply the right treatment at the right time on the right people.

"About four years after my stroke I was in a clinical trial for CIMT with Dr. Taub, who developed this therapy. At the time, his clinic in Alabama was one of the only places to get CIMT. Now it's available around the country. The treatment was very intense and very time-consuming. It helped my arm and shoulder a little bit, but not my hand. I'm glad I tried it, but it was frustrating. For me, I noticed a small improvement. But most survivors with less paralysis see large improvements. Every stroke is different, so it could be an option for you." — David

A Tip from Dr. Mike

"The human brain is one of the most wondrous and advanced entities in the universe. Each one is complex, and each stroke is different. The professionals treating you are experts in their fields. However, I also tell my patients this: 'Only *you* are the true expert of *you*. You are the only one who knows what it's truly like to be in your body with this brain. Throughout this process, become the expert of what *you* need for an optimal recovery.'"

32. How can technology help with recovery of physical function?

Dr. Stoykov: I'm a fan of low-tech technology. There are a few things you can do to train the brain or trick it into working better. One is called *mirror therapy*. You place a mirror between the two sides of your body, with the mirror facing your good arm, and you put the affected arm behind the mirror so that you don't see it. Then when you look at the mirror, you see the movement of your good arm, but your brain thinks it's the affected arm moving. You're tricking the brain into thinking the affected arm is making normal movements. You'd want to try this with an occupational therapist first to learn if it's right for you and how to do it at home.

Another thing you can try with a therapist is called *bilateral priming*. I use something called an Exsurgo bilateral priming device, but I call it a *flapper*. It's a device where each hand goes between two plates that are connected together so that the stronger wrist moves the weaker wrist in and out at the same time. I have my patients use it for 15 to 20 minutes before they do their occupational therapy, and I've seen a big difference between those who've done the bilateral priming and those who haven't.

Dr. Gillen: We use bowling or tennis video games on consoles like Wii and Xbox to help people work on balance or limb function. It's very motivating to people, even older adults. The Kinect device for the Xbox doesn't even use controllers, so it's like virtual reality. And it's commercially available to everyone.

There are various apps on smartphones that help with stroke recovery. For example, you can use apps to track home exercise programs. There's also a whole emerging world of *telehealth* or *telerehabilitation* that lets you consult with a therapist via FaceTime or Skype if you can't actually come to a therapy session.

> *"There was very little technology available when I was in therapy, but the Wii was new. I really liked that the therapist used something fun to help with strength and balance, and that proved helpful as I was able to use it at home too. The occupational therapist used Velcro or an ACE bandage to keep the remote in my right hand. Having fun can help you get through this process. Have fun. Laugh. Smile. It's great medicine."* — David

A Tip from Dr. Mike

"Doing something fun is one behavioral element of cognitive behavioral therapy. When we're feeling low, it can be helpful to choose an activity that brings us pleasure, like playing a game with someone, taking a bath, or watching a funny movie. When we smile and laugh, the brain releases neurochemicals that improve our mood. This lightness goes a long way—especially when we're going through a difficult time. Another simple trick from the Buddhist tradition that has been shown to have powerful neurochemical effects in the brain: put a *Mona Lisa* smile on your face through everything you do. Smile when you wake up. Smile through that difficult physical therapy session. Smile when you're having a hard day as a caretaker. It actually tricks the brain into thinking it's happy, which can release feel-good hormones and promote actions that lead to real, spontaneous smiles."

Dr. Page: There's a new device called the MyoPro that's being successfully administered through the VA and is increasingly being covered by insurance. This electronic brace, created by a company called Myomo, is a *myoelectric device,* meaning it detects and amplifies the electric signals from the muscles to help the patient move. That's a really exciting development because it means someone can get a brace fitted to the affected arm, and then use this device to help him or her do things at home, like flip a light switch, turn a key in a lock, get up out of a chair, or pick up a laundry basket. The device is affixed to the arm, so it's portable, and it gives patients the extra help they need to perform valued activities.

33. What can stroke survivors do to make one-handed life easier?

Dr. Page: An occupational therapist can help you identify adaptations. You might have to learn things like one-handed shoe tying or writing with the nondominant hand. There are tools like one-handed can openers, reachers, and sock aids. One of our jobs as therapists is to educate stroke survivors on the use of this equipment to help them be successful and independent. The exact tools depend on the patient and where the impairments are, but there are adaptations available. Magazines like *StrokeSmart* have lots of advertisements in the back for one-handed tools to help stroke survivors.

"Adapting to being one-handed was challenging. I worked on improving, but I had to work on adapting too. For example, I now have an automatic light that turns on when I walk in the room. I also have a magnetic doorstop for my front door that helps when I'm bringing in groceries. The lid of my trash can opens automatically when my hand waves over it. Work on strengthening your abilities as much as you can, and then use the tools where you need them." — David

A Tip from Dr. Mike

"Every human being has strengths and weaknesses. If you've had a stroke, these strengths and weaknesses may have changed. An approach that focuses on your strengths can help you be more successful in your life. So work with your strengths while simultaneously addressing your weaknesses. Stay honest, open, and willing through this process. What are your strengths today? What are the weaknesses you'd like to address?"

● ● ● ● ●

TAKEAWAY POINTS:

The upper extremity is often slowest to recover because its movements are so complex, requiring a large area in the brain to control it. Keep using the affected hand and arm as much as possible in safe ways. Stimulate them with sensory feedback and continue to stretch. Watch out for learned nonuse.

Constraint-induced therapy can be effective for people with some movement in the wrist and fingers.

There are tools to make one-handed living easier. Talk to your occupational therapist to find out which ones are best for you, and also search online for one-handed products.

CHAPTER 6

RECOVERING YOUR COGNITION

A stroke damages the brain, impacting both the body and the mind. Unfortunately, about a third of stroke survivors may experience significant changes in their thinking skills—things like memory, attention, and reasoning. They may face challenges with interpreting what they see. These impairments can negatively affect safety and independence. We continued our talk with occupational therapy expert Dr. Glen Gillen to bring you information on the effects of strokes on cognition and perception. Learn what you can do to speed recovery of these critical functions of the brain for you or your loved one.

34. What are cognition and perception?

Dr. Gillen: They are two different things. *Cognition* includes all the **mental functions** that support everyday living. *Perception* is our ability to **take in information** through the senses and interpret it. We usually take these things for granted, because we don't think about them when they're working. It's only when things become impaired, when we can't go on autopilot anymore, that we become aware of these mental processes.

For example, if you're going to the grocery store, the first thing you do is get into your vehicle. You have to remember how to work the vehicle—we call that *procedural memory*—and that is a cognitive function. The next thing you need to do is remember the way to the grocery store. We call that *way finding*, and that's a cognitive function. If, on the way to the grocery store, your usual route is disrupted by a closed road, you then need to *problem solve* to find another route, and that's another cognitive function. Once you're in the grocery store, you need to *remember* your list of groceries, another cognitive function.

A grocery store is a stimulating environment, so you need to be able to *sustain attention* on the task at hand and not be distracted by whatever is going on around you. That's another cognitive function. When you check out, you need to do *calculations* related to your money management—making sure you have enough money, getting the correct change, and so on—and that's another cognitive function. Throughout the "simple" task of grocery shopping, multiple cognitive functions are required.

35. How are cognition and perception affected by a stroke?

Dr. Gillen: Unfortunately, they're very commonly impaired by a stroke, and these impairments limit our ability to engage in everyday tasks.

Attention deficits are highly prevalent and also long lasting. After a stroke you might lose your ability to sustain your attention over time or to attend to items selectively without being distracted.

Memory functions of different types tend to become impaired. Short-term memory, or *working memory*, is required for you to keep things in mind as you work with them. Some people lose their *long-term memory*, becoming unable to remember things that happened prior to the stroke. They also can't hold on to new memories.

A major impact of a stroke is the inability to be **aware of the deficit** you have. That's a scary combination—cognitive deficits that might lead to safety concerns, and not even being aware that you have those deficits. We spend a lot of time evaluating awareness of deficits before we treat them.

Perceptual deficits are both fascinating and highly frustrating. There are people who have the ability to see, but they can't recognize an object in front of them. That's called *agnosia*. Some people may lose their *color perception*, which is less extreme but can affect their quality of life. Other people lose their *depth perception*. So if they're reaching for an object like a glass, they might reach past it, or if they're stepping up a staircase, they might misperceive the height of the step and trip. Another common impairment after a stroke is what we call *left neglect*. Left neglect is a one-sided attention disorder, meaning people don't pay attention to information on the left side, even though their vision is fine. They read only half the page, eat the food on only half of their plate, and talk to people on only one side of the table at family meal.

These perceptual deficits after a stroke can be quite devastating if they're not picked up. But if they are noticed, there's a lot we can do about them, so it's important that stroke survivors get specific evaluations in the area of cognition and perception from their rehab team.

Visual deficits are also prevalent after a stroke, depending on where the stroke occurred. It's common to experience *loss of acuity*, so even if you wore glasses before, your glasses might not offer the same correction that they did prior to the stroke. People also have issues related to *double vision* after a stroke. The other big one is *visual field loss*, where people have blind spots in their eyes. There are occupational therapists, ophthalmologists, and neuro-ophthalmologists for whom these visual deficits become a specialty. The key is to seek out these vision specialists so you can get a comprehensive evaluation to figure out what your exact visual deficit is. The good news is that they have techniques that can get your vision to where it's more comfortable for you, if not back to normal.

36. Who can help with cognitive recovery?

Dr. Gillen: There are many professionals involved in cognitive rehabilitation because it has such a lasting impact on a patient's life. Each of these professionals makes a unique contribution to the area of cognitive rehabilitation.

People should seek out the services of **occupational therapists** if their cognitive deficits are having an impact on their everyday lives.

Your everyday life could include tasks as simple as taking care of your body, dressing yourself in the morning, or bathing yourself. Or it could include more complex tasks, such as parenting, going to school, or working. Occupational therapy can help with these areas of your life.

Neuropsychologists diagnose cognitive deficits with detailed assessments, and now they're also moving into interventions related to cognitive rehab. If you want to reenter your community, return to school, or return to work—anything beyond a schedule that's the same every day—it's important to get a neuropsychological assessment.

Speech-language pathologists also look at cognition, specifically as it relates to communication—understanding, speaking, reading, or writing.

Author's note: Many stroke survivors wonder why they're seeing a speech-language pathologist when they can "talk just fine." However, cognitive problems nearly always have some impact on communication. A person with a cognitive-communication disorder may have difficulty paying attention to a conversation, staying on topic, remembering information, responding accurately, understanding jokes, or following directions. These problems can have a negative impact on social situations, as well as on daily routines and responsibilities. Speech therapy can help to improve communication by targeting the underlying cognitive skills.

37. How can therapy help people deal with problems with cognition and perception?

Dr. Gillen: It's a two-phase approach. First is the idea of **awareness building,** and it starts from day one and continues throughout the rehabilitation process. What is striking about awareness is that most patients are aware of their motor deficits but not their cognitive deficits. If I walk into a room, the first thing they'll say to me is, "I can't walk anymore. I can't use my right arm." Rarely will people say early on after a stroke, "I'm forgetting things," or "I can't attend to things on the left side of my body," or "I'm distracted."

Self-awareness of deficits is essential for safety, and it's essential for stroke recovery. We have had some people with severe perceptual deficits tell us they're going to drive home from the hospital, and that would be disastrous. People fall when they are in the rehab unit because they're not aware that they can't stand up on their own. You have to be aware of what you can and can't do. Once you know you have a problem and understand how it affects your life, you can set realistic goals and start to work on them.

The next phase, after awareness, is **strategy training**. Despite having a cognitive deficit or perceptual deficit, we can circumvent it by using various strategies. To buy into using a strategy, people have to be aware of their deficits first. So it's awareness training, and then it's strategy training to try to circumvent the impairment.

38. Cognitive, perceptual, and communication problems aren't always visible to people on the street. How can stroke survivors with these problems best interact with others when they have an invisible disability?

Dr. Gillen: In many cases, people have a combination of motor and cognitive deficits, so it's clear to the person you're interacting with that something has happened. If you have a cognitive, perceptual, or communication deficit but no motor deficit—no limp, weak hand, or something that you can see—it becomes problematic because people don't know how to interact with you.

It's really important to empower the stroke survivor to **take responsibility to make other people feel comfortable**. Going back to that idea of awareness, we use the term *online awareness* or *emergent awareness*, which means that you're understanding in real time when an interaction's not going right. For these situations we coach people to say things like "I'm having trouble understanding you; can we go to another part of the hallway where there are fewer people around?" "I'm going to ask you to repeat that a couple of times because I have trouble remembering things," or "Do you mind if I take out my phone and jot notes on this conversation, or take out my daily planner?" When the stroke survivor takes the lead, it makes the person whom they're interacting with feel more comfortable with the interaction. Otherwise the person can misperceive that the stroke survivor is not paying attention or is not interested in the social interaction.

We use those strategies a lot when people go back to work environments. You don't have to disclose that you had a stroke, but your co-workers might misinterpret your invisible disability and think you're a poor employee or you're not as invested as the rest of them. So it really falls on the stroke survivor to make the other person involved in the interaction feel comfortable and understand what the deficit is.

39. What can family members do to help their loved ones with cognitive problems?

Dr. Gillen: Just as we have to modify the physical environment to be safe, we also have to **modify the social environment** at home. That might mean more education for the family to help them understand that the stroke survivor may comprehend but may take longer to react. They have to speak more slowly, or wait longer for a response. If somebody is distractible and has an attention deficit, a family meal can be fun but also very frustrating because people are talking over each other and there are multiple conversations going on. So you try to **limit the distractions** to make the person feel engaged and part of the family unit.

When a stroke survivor is trying to communicate a thought, we instinctively want to finish his or her sentence and move on, but that's not always going to help the person. We are natural helpers; we want to help our loved ones. But overhelping might do a disservice. Sometimes we have to **give stroke survivors some time** and let them figure things out for themselves, which feels good for them, rather than jump in to help right away.

For memory problems, we can use very low-tech solutions like placing sticky notes with reminders of what has to be done in key places around the house, such as next to the bed, on the kitchen counter, or on the bathroom mirror. We can also use higher-tech solutions like alarm reminders on our phones. We use things like memory books and diaries all the time for people to remind themselves about their appointments, or that they need to make an appointment. Families can support their loved ones in being more independent by using **strategies** like these.

◇◇◇

A stroke survivor says, "I'm so sensitive to noise now. It's overwhelming to go out to a restaurant or the mall. Why is this, and what can I do about it?"

Dr. Gillen: It's a problem with *selective attention*. If you're walking in a mall, there are so many conversations going on around you. Someone who hasn't had a stroke can focus on the person they're shopping with and screen out all that irrelevant background noise. After a stroke, that becomes very difficult.

There are a couple of things to try. The first is to **go during off-peak times**. Go to the mall or to a restaurant when it's not going to be the busiest, such as on a Friday evening at the mall or during an early-bird special in a restaurant. You also need to control your own environment in terms of distractions. For example, turn off the TV or radio when talking, because what's background noise for some becomes overwhelming for the stroke survivor. You can also try **wearing noise-canceling headphones** without music playing through them to decrease the distraction.

◇◇◇

40. How can technology help with cognitive problems after a stroke?

Dr. Gillen: In the cognitive domain, a smartphone really can become a cognitive *prosthesis*—a device that helps when the body or brain isn't working right. We can set up alerts and reminders to take pills or go to an appointment. We can make to-do lists to keep ourselves organized. Technology is an integral part of our day-to-day lives, so everyone can use it to help with memory and organization.

Using Technology to Improve Cognition from Megan

Technology can be an amazing tool to help stroke survivors function better in daily life. There's no shame in using a tool or strategy to help—nearly everyone today relies on a paper or digital calendar to remember appointments. Our lives are simply too complicated for anyone to keep everything in his or her head. Your smartphone is already filled with tools you can use to help with cognition. These are the apps you'll find on an iPhone, but there are similar apps on Android phones:

- **Calendar:** Enter future appointments and create alerts to remind you when it's time to get ready and time to leave. You can also enter the things you've done each day so you can look back to know when something happened.

- **Maps:** Get turn-by-turn directions to your destination so you won't get lost. Drop a pin on the map to remember where you parked. Explore walking, biking, and public transit routes if you're not driving.

- **Camera:** Take pictures of the things you do and see during the day to help you remember. When someone shows you something you'd like to look into further, snap a photo so you won't forget.

- **Contacts:** Add photos to your address book to reference when you can't remember someone's name. Add birthdays, family members, and notes about how you know each person.

- **Clock:** Alarms aren't just for waking up in the morning. Set alarms for times throughout the day to remind you to take your medication, do your exercises, or drink enough water—whatever you regularly forget to do.

- **Calculator:** To calculate tips or divide checks, just use the calculator.

- **Notes and Reminders:** Make shopping lists and add to them as you notice you've run out of something. Set reminders for when it's time to pay bills (or better yet, automate your payments so you won't have to think about them).

- **Voice Memos:** If typing is a problem, record your spoken notes or send voice-based text messages. Use the built-in dictation feature on your keyboard to turn your voice into printed words in any app.

- **Find My Friends:** Share your GPS location with your family members so they won't worry about where you've gone. Specialized tracking apps are available for those with a history of wandering off.

- **Health:** Track your blood pressure, steps, and other exercise goals. Add a wearable fitness band for closer monitoring of your heart rate, sleep, and activity. Physical exercise may be the best therapy for cognitive problems as it increases blood flow to the brain.

The most challenging part of using an app or strategy might be remembering to use it when you need it! Find the tools that work best for you; then practice using them over and over until they become a habit.

◇◇

A stroke survivor asks, "What about brain-training games? Do they help?"

Dr. Gillen: When they're used in isolation as the whole therapy, I'm not a fan. We have to consider *generalization*. What tends to happen is you become better at playing the game, but does that brain training allow you to be able to balance your checkbook or to search the web to find the cheapest airline tickets? Most studies have shown that you will improve on the game or activities that are very similar to the game, but not necessarily on other activities.

That being said, I'm a fan of an active brain, so if the games are done in conjunction with a full rehab program and are only a side activity, then there's absolutely nothing wrong with them and I would encourage their use. If people are motivated by a program like Lumosity, that's great, but it can't be the only thing. It's not going to be the change agent for people, but it's probably better than watching TV.

◇◇

• • • • •

Takeaway Points:

Impairments in cognition and perception are very common after a stroke. This can include problems with attention, memory, and processing what is seen. Stroke survivors may not even be aware they have these problems, which puts safety at risk.

Cognitive therapy can be performed by an occupational therapist, speech-language pathologist, or neuropsychologist. Therapy for cognition first builds self-awareness, then trains the patient to use strategies to deal with the problems.

Cognitive and perceptual problems are often invisible disabilities. Stroke survivors can learn to recognize when their disabilities are creating problems, then take the lead on using a strategy or educating others.

Family members may need to modify how they interact with a stroke survivor with cognitive impairments. Limit distractions, speak slower, be patient, and use strategies.

Use technology to help with memory and organization and to keep the brain active.

CHAPTER 7

RECOVERING YOUR COMMUNICATION

Another cognitive function that can become impaired after a stroke is communication. Losing your ability to communicate your thoughts and ideas clearly can be absolutely devastating. The most important thing to remember is that speech is a skill, just like walking, that doesn't change who you are when it's gone. You are still an intelligent, unique person.

Communication problems after a stroke are especially near and dear to our hearts. David couldn't speak at all after his stroke, and he was fortunate to have countless hours of speech therapy to help him recover. One of David's speech therapists was Dr. Jacqueline Hinckley, associate professor emeritus of speech-language pathology at the University of South Florida. Another influential person in David's life was the world-renowned speech-language pathologist Dr. Audrey Holland, an aphasia researcher, advocate, and the Regents' professor emeritus of speech, language, and hearing sciences at the University of Arizona. They kindly share their expertise on communication disorders with you now.

41. What kinds of communication problems can happen after a stroke?

Author's note: There are three main types of communication problems that can happen after damage to the brain. Two affect speech, and the other affects language. **Speech** is the sounds we produce to communicate, and **language** is the words we say. You may have one, two, or all three problems.

Dysarthria is a type of communication problem that causes **slurred speech**. There are a few simple strategies to improve the clarity of your speech: slow down, speak a bit louder, and *overarticulate* (exaggerate your mouth movements). A speech-language pathologist can recommend specific exercises based on your symptoms to help improve slurred speech.

There's another kind of speech problem called *apraxia*. Apraxia makes it hard to coordinate or **sequence the movements** of the muscles in the mouth when speaking. Apraxia nearly always happens alongside *aphasia*, the main communication problem that affects language after a stroke. Aphasia affects about a third of all stroke survivors. Aphasia and apraxia are treated together to help stroke survivors communicate more effectively.

42. What is aphasia?

Dr. Hinckley: Aphasia is the **disruption of language** after a stroke. When I say "language," I mean understanding what people say to you and being able to say what you mean, as well as reading and writing.

Try to imagine being in a country where people speak a different language. You don't understand it, can't speak it, and can't read it or write it either. You can look around and understand what's going on, but you have a barrier of communication. People with aphasia have that kind of problem. It may be that they can't say or understand anything, or it may be as if they know a little bit of the language but not as much as they would like.

Unfortunately, many times in our society we equate the ability to speak with intelligence, so people treat those with aphasia or other speech problems differently. **People with aphasia still have their intelligence**, but they're not able to convey it through the normal language channels. That's very difficult for people to understand. I've even heard people with aphasia say, "Gosh, I'm not smart anymore."

That's simply not true. It may be hard to understand and to communicate, but aphasia affects only your command of language, not your intelligence.

43. Are all cases of aphasia the same, or are there different types of aphasia?

Dr. Hinckley: There are **many different types of aphasia** with various names to reflect the different impairment profiles people can have. Some people with aphasia have much greater difficulty with understanding speech than others (*Wernicke's aphasia*), some have much greater difficulty saying what they want to say (*Broca's aphasia*), and some people have difficulty with everything (*global aphasia*). Similarly, there are differences for reading and writing abilities. These problems can be combined in different ways and to varying degrees, depending on which parts of the brain were affected by the stroke.

Dr. Holland: I have **never met two people whose aphasia is exactly alike.** Aphasia doesn't involve just language; it also involves motivation, attitude, and energy. Those factors are not all the same for all people. When you've met one person with aphasia, you've met one person with aphasia.

When you explain aphasia to others, you should be very specific to the particular needs of the person with aphasia. You can say, "He has trouble talking. He also has trouble understanding, particularly if you talk too fast or too much. He gets tired easily. He can read very well, but he can't write."

"My aphasia was really, really bad. I could hardly speak at all in the first couple of years. When I was 12, I went to Dr. Hinckley, and she is an amazing speech-language pathologist. She taught me ways to communicate through means besides talking, and she engaged me in things I was interested in, so I wanted to communicate, and I made a lot of progress. Wherever you are with your speech, keep working on it. Word by word. Day by day." — David

A Tip from Dr. Mike

"Being interested in a topic improves attention span and can make a task enjoyable. Explore topics you like to keep yourself engaged in the recovery process. If you like football, read the sports section out loud or talk with a friend about last night's game. If you like art, go to a museum with someone and have a conversation about your favorite exhibit. Just because something is therapeutic doesn't mean you can't make it interesting. The recipe for a happy life is to fill it with pleasure, passion, and purpose."

44. What does recovery look like for somebody with aphasia?

Dr. Holland: You can expect to see the biggest gains within the first two or three months in the period of spontaneous recovery, but recovery can go on and on for many years following a stroke. It's important that people who have had a stroke and their families don't give up hope, and that they continue to be resilient and optimistic about the ultimate long-term recovery. I'm not willing to make a prediction about how much better someone with aphasia is going to get, but it is pretty clear that when you have aphasia, you're never going to be more aphasic than you are the first day you have the disorder. There certainly is hope, and there is help.

45. How can speech therapy help people with communication problems?

Dr. Hinckley: Therapy should be oriented toward **helping people get back to doing the activities that are most important to them.** That is essential, not only because they want to get back to doing those things, but also because therapy can be most effective when it's embedded in what's motivating to stroke survivors. The way our brains change can be enhanced if we're doing things that are meaningful to us.

We often hear "Use it or lose it." Another principle of neuroplasticity is "Use it and improve it." If the therapy is very directly focused on what the patients want to do, then they're going to keep doing it more throughout the day and across days. When they get more practice and repetition, they're likely to improve more.

Also, we have quite a number of therapy approaches that have been researched, so we know what the probable outcomes will be. If we use these *evidence-based* therapies, and they're matched properly to a person, then we increase the likelihood that good improvement is going to be made. In addition, most of the research we have for the effectiveness of aphasia therapy is based on stroke survivors who are beyond the first six months of recovery, so we know people continue to improve with therapy.

46. How does group therapy compare to individual therapy?

Dr. Hinckley: Group therapy has some very nice advantages. When you're in a group situation, you are practicing your social communication skills. You're trying to get your message across to people who may or may not understand it, so you have lots of opportunities to problem-solve with support. In addition, the psychological and social support of being with people who are facing a similar circumstance is very encouraging. You might see somebody else with aphasia using a communication strategy that you haven't tried before, and it might work for you.

Individual therapy, since it's tailored specifically to you, gives you dedicated time to practice the specific skills you want to improve that are harder to work on in a group setting, like reading and writing. The best situation is to have a **combination of both individual and group therapy.**

"I co-founded Aphasia Recovery Connection. We have a group on Facebook to connect people with aphasia. Not everyone has a stroke or aphasia center nearby. Our group is available 24/7 online, and it's filled with people who really understand what you're experiencing. Being surrounded by people going through the same thing can help you remember that you're not alone."
— David

A Tip from Dr. Mike

"Watch out for *terminal uniqueness*—the belief that the situation you're in is unlike anything faced by anyone else. It affects stroke survivors and loved ones alike, and it leads to isolation, depression, and anxiety. Cure terminal uniqueness by putting yourself in situations where you're not the only one. Remember: there are millions of stroke survivors in this world. Go meet some of them! At Aphasia Recovery Connection, for example, you'll be surrounded by other survivors and family members. By hearing and relating to other people's shared experiences, feelings are normalized. This leads to connection, hope, and faith."

47. What can family members do to help loved ones with aphasia?

Dr. Holland: The most important thing for family members is to **learn to communicate** with their loved ones with aphasia and to learn the techniques that are involved in what is called *supported communication*. This is where you change your own language style to make the person with aphasia better able to understand. By using paper, gestures, and specific questions, it is also easier for the person with aphasia to express him- or herself. It's bigger than just using picture boards, though that helps some people; supported communication is about changing your communication style to reveal the competence of the person with aphasia. For example, asking the person with aphasia to verify what he meant by something, learning what his strongest communication modality is (gesturing, writing, drawing, speaking), reminding him that he might try writing something, or giving him some written choices to pick from. It's really a strength-oriented approach, using what the person can do instead of focusing on what they can't.

Also, it's important for families to understand fully that aphasia is a language disorder. It doesn't mean that cognitive abilities in general are affected. Knowing that the person's mind is all right may be the most important thing early on. Then the families have to understand that this is a long process and that recovery will go on. A lot of recovery comes from the brain settling down, so it isn't all related to therapy; it's also related to time.

Families can also look for things that their loved ones are still able to do with or without language. Communication isn't all just speech; it can be holding your hand as a way to say "I love you." It can be things that are gestural or written—all modes of communication count.

Communication Tips for Aphasia from Megan

Aphasia can be extremely frustrating, both for the stroke survivor and the communication partner. By making some adjustments in how you speak, you can help to ease that frustration. Here are a few small things you can do that will make a big difference when talking to a person with aphasia:

- Share the burden of communication, recognizing that it's not the problem only of the person with aphasia. Be patient, and allow plenty of time for communication.

- Say "I know you know" to acknowledge that the person with aphasia is intelligent with ideas he or she wants to express but can't.

- Speak in short, simple sentences with an expressive voice, but don't shout, talk down, or use baby talk. Think of talking to someone who doesn't speak English as a first language.

- Use writing, gestures, drawings, and body language to supplement verbal communication. Point to objects or use pictures. Keep paper and pen handy to write down key words.

- Ask yes/no questions (Do you want tea?), include options in your questions (Do you want tea or coffee?), or offer written choices (tea, coffee, juice) to make it easier for the person with aphasia to express an opinion.

- Ask questions one at a time, starting with general questions and then moving toward specifics (Is it about a person? Is it a family member? Is it Karen?). Keep in mind that a yes/no response may not be completely reliable, so it's okay to double-check.

- Eliminate distractions and background noise, speaking in a quiet environment. One-on-one interaction is usually better than a large group.

- Repeat what you think you understood to make sure it's correct. Don't pretend you understand if you don't.

- Ask the person if he wants you to answer for him or fill in his words when he's struggling. Some people appreciate the help, while others would rather speak for themselves.

Remember that it's okay to give up if things get too frustrating. You can agree to come back to an idea later when it might come out more easily.

Dr. Hinckley: We need to be patient. Those of us who do not have aphasia are used to taking turns in conversation in one second or less, but when you have aphasia, it's not uncommon to need 10 or 20 seconds to get going on the message. That's 10 or 20 times longer than we're all used to waiting. That is very hard for people to do. I'll ask caregivers to count just three to five seconds after they finish speaking before speaking again. For some people, even waiting that long seems like an eternity. It's very hard for them to wait, but they need to practice it to give the person time.

Many people are not comfortable with silence. There is a lot of silence with aphasia, so we need to do things to help ourselves be more comfortable with silence, to feel that it's okay and not a bad thing. Mindfulness or meditation may be a way to help with this. Sometimes people with aphasia get tired. They're working so hard with all these words that are coming at them or that they're trying to say. It's important to have these quiet times. You can sit quietly on a park bench and look at the beauty of nature, and just share the space in silence. Those things are very important too.

◇◇◇

A caregiver asks, "If you can tell when a person with aphasia wants to say something, and you think you know what the person wants to say, should you help the person with the words?"

Dr. Holland: I don't have the answer to that. That answer lies with the person with aphasia. What works for one person will not work for somebody else. When a family member says, "What should I do? I don't know if I should give him the word or not." I always say, "I'm not the one to ask. Ask him what he wants you to do. And he'll tell you—either 'Leave me alone; I want to struggle with it,' or 'I can use the help.'"

The person with aphasia should be given every opportunity to feel his own strength and to be empowered. There are three sources of expertise, sort of like a three-legged stool. There are the academics or clinicians who have studied aphasia and work with it; there are the family members who live with the people and know them well; and most important there's the people with aphasia themselves—the true experts in what they need because they live it. You need all three legs for the stool to stand.

Dr. Hinckley: Family members face a high-wire act in terms of balancing their desire and need to help with encouraging independence. That's not easy. The thing is to talk about it and work with the person with aphasia to find the right balance, not just decide unilaterally what you think should be done, because the person with aphasia probably has his own opinion too and it should be taken into account.

◇◇

48. What can people with aphasia do to improve their communication at home?

Dr. Holland: They can do things daily that get them communicating with others. Therapy doesn't happen just in a room with a professional, but every day out in the world. The famous psychiatrist Fritz Perls said, "The end of therapy is when everything becomes therapeutic."

Another important thing is to get the person with aphasia involved with other people who have aphasia, and to do this early on. It's a terrific support to surround yourself with other people with aphasia, because they understand what it's like. They are people who live with the problem, and they are incredibly helpful to each other. Getting involved with an aphasia community is one of the most potent, long-term treatments for aphasia that we have.

Dr. Hinckley: Yes, it's very important for the person with aphasia to seek out aphasia or stroke support groups. The National Aphasia Association lists programs by region so people can find a place where they can go to get support, even though it's not formal therapy. That support is more than just social support (although that's critical too); it also means you're getting out of the house, you're being active, and you're getting back to doing activities. All of that is very important to continue improving.

As I've mentioned before, an important principle of changing and improving your brain is "Use it or lose it." So it's very important to **stay active and engaged.** I have always told my patients that there is one guaranteed way to stop making progress if you have aphasia after a stroke: sit on the couch, watch TV, and don't do anything else. If that's your day, then you probably will stop improving because you're not engaging your brain and using your communication skills in any meaningful way.

So the first thing is to stay active, but that's probably more easily said than done after a stroke. I would suggest people find something that they can do, something accessible to them and something very important to them, and just start doing it. **Get out into the community.** Finding an aphasia group or finding friends, neighbors, and family members who can help get you out so you continue doing things is probably the most important step.

In ideal circumstances, a speech-language pathologist will set up some kind of exercise program that you will be able to continue to do at home. Technology provides us with a lot of different options as there are now so many **apps and practice programs** available. Ideally, the speech-language pathologist will help you find the app or software that's going to be a good fit for you, and help you set it up.

49. How can technology help people with aphasia?

Dr. Hinckley: Just in the last few years we've had an explosion of apps and technology available for aphasia. There are some tools that are designed for people to create or use stored messages so that when they go out into the community—to order at a restaurant, for example—they can communicate better. Apps that do that are probably my favorites because they are combining the smarts of the technology with the support of helping the person get out into the community and actually interact with others.

There are many software programs and apps that are designed for drill work, such as practicing spelling or understanding words. These can help people practice specific skills, but they shouldn't be used to the exclusion of having conversations with family members or other people. That's a concern that we have to be aware of with technology—people being glued to their phones or sitting in front of a computer all day.

Dr. Holland: Technology is a booming industry, and it can offer so much for people with aphasia. It runs the gamut, from speech-generating devices to *teletherapy* (working with a therapist via a video chat) to online support groups like the Aphasia Recovery Connection.

Choosing good apps and sticking with them is more important than downloading hundreds of apps. Once you find apps that you like, keep using them! And don't forget about the apps and features that are built right into your phone or device, like having text read aloud or taking photos. Learning to use those is just as important as learning to use the apps specialized for aphasia. It's also okay to have apps for fun. I'm addicted to Words with Friends. It's a game like Scrabble that you can play at any level, and it's a language activity. Apps like that are just fun, and the importance of that shouldn't be discounted.

Using Technology to Improve Communication from Megan

Technology can help stroke survivors with aphasia in three ways: to connect, to communicate, and to improve.

- **Connect:** Phones have always allowed us to talk to people far away, but with video chats through Skype, FaceTime, or Google, people with aphasia can communicate better by using gestures, writing, and facial expressions. Sending text messages and e-mail allows people more time to compose their thoughts, look up their words, and respond. Social media keeps stroke survivors connected with family and friends far away and makes it easy to meet new people who understand strokes and aphasia. Joining an online support group like Aphasia Recovery Connection can lead to more communication opportunities.

- **Communicate:** Tools and strategies that supplement or replace verbal communication are called *augmentative and alternative communication* (AAC). AAC can be low-tech like a pad of paper or a picture communication book, or it can be high-tech like an iPad. There are many AAC apps available to help people with aphasia to communicate. They are not a cure, but they can help if the app is carefully selected and customized and the person is trained. Lingraphica offers some free AAC apps as well as dedicated AAC devices for aphasia. The built-in Camera, Photos, Maps, Calendar, and Notes apps can also be used for communication, along with whiteboard apps for quickly writing or drawing messages. Accessibility features like voice dictation and text to speech can also help with reading and writing. (For more ideas on using the built-in apps on your phone, refer back to the "Using Technology to Improve Cognition" box on page 66.)

- **Improve:** Using therapy apps and software can be a great way to increase the intensity of your practice. The research evidence shows us that computerized therapy can be very effective in helping people with aphasia improve, even years after a stroke. Keep recovery going by working on your own or with a partner at home. Look for apps designed specifically for adults with aphasia and based on therapy activities proven to work, like those by Tactus Therapy. Ask your speech-language pathologist to help you find the right activities to challenge you.

◇◇

A stroke survivor asks, "Does watching TV help with language improvements?"

Dr. Hinckley: One way to think about this question is to ask, "If you watch TV in Spanish, will you learn Spanish?" If all you do is watch a TV program, then the answer is probably no. But if watching a program is combined with talking about it or reading about it, then it can help as part of those larger activities. Simply sitting and watching TV is a very passive activity, and our brain needs to be active to improve, so it's not a very helpful activity on its own.

Of course we all have our favorite programs, and it's a good thing to watch a program that you enjoy. Try it with the closed-captioning on to see if that's helpful. Many people with aphasia find that it helps, though others find it to be an unhelpful distraction. However, even with reading the captions, sitting at home and watching TV all day is still not a good idea.

◇◇

50. Does a person with a communication problem have the right to make his or her own decisions?

Dr. Hinckley: Absolutely. The only time somebody does not make his own decisions is when he is legally deemed *incompetent* to make those decisions, and that usually has to do with not being able to think clearly or reason things out. **Aphasia alone should not prevent somebody from being able to make his or her own decisions.** However, it is going to mean that the person with aphasia may need some support to understand any legal or technical documents. If there are financial issues, the person might need a little help in understanding, but once he does, he has the right to make decisions about it.

The Aphasia Institute has a series of booklets that have pictographs and simplified language to support people with aphasia when talking about different complex issues with social workers and others. That support can be very helpful.

• • • • •

TAKEAWAY POINTS:

Communication problems are common after a stroke. They can be problems with speech (dysarthria or apraxia) or language (aphasia). Aphasia is a language disorder that can impair speaking, understanding, reading, and writing in varying degrees in each person. It is *not* a problem with intelligence.

Speech therapy can help people with aphasia to recover. Group therapy and individual therapy are both helpful, especially when evidence-based treatments are used.

Family members can help best by learning to adapt their own communication styles to support the person with aphasia.

- Be patient. Allow the person more time to process and respond.

- Show respect for the person's intelligence, which might be hidden by his or her language problem.

- Enjoy each other in silence, and find new ways to communicate.

Ask the person with aphasia if he wants you to help or speak for him. He's the expert in what he needs or wants.

Staying active and engaged in the community and in life is the best therapy. Don't sit at home, watching TV all day. Join an aphasia group to get out of the house and meet others who understand.

Use technology to help your recovery. Practicing exercises by using apps or software can intensify your rehab and help with neuroplasticity. Use communication apps to help when you're out in the community, and join an online support group like the Aphasia Recovery Connection to connect with others.

People with aphasia still have the right to make their own decisions, but they may need extra support.

CHAPTER 8

RECOVERING
THE RIGHT WAY

If you want to achieve your best recovery, it's not enough just to attend your therapy sessions. A few hours a week won't cut it—you have to do more. Combining good therapists with the right approaches applied intensively can help you beat the odds and get better faster. Several of our experts weighed in to help us understand the best ways to approach therapy and rehabilitation, and what to do when it seems like progress has stopped or when hope starts to fade.

51. How can stroke survivors maximize the time they spend in therapy?

Dr. Roth: You have to think about therapy in broad terms. Formal therapy is provided by the physical, occupational, and speech therapists and other rehab professionals, but really the issue is not just therapy. The real issue is **activation, activity, and engagement**. It's obviously ideal to have as much of the professional involvement as reasonable or possible, but oftentimes family members and patients themselves, if they have the motivation and the capability, can do some of the exercises.

We urge all of our staff to **provide home exercises** to their patients, and **teach the family members** if they're available. But we also urge the patients themselves to keep active. Sometimes simple things like exercising the fingers, moving the arms, practicing standing up, or transferring between the bed and the wheelchair can be valuable. For people with communication problems, practicing talking and reading aloud can be very valuable.

We try to **minimize the downtime**. It really is "use it or lose it." A lot of the disability actually derives from just not paying attention to or not using the limb or the language. Ignoring it actually makes it weaker.

"It is important to be rested to be our best for our rehab sessions. They are valuable. And they don't last forever. Be on time. Be rested. Be ready to work. This willing and positive attitude is one of the most important parts of recovery." — David

A Tip from Dr. Mike

"One of the best predictors of recovery in general is how willing and motivated a patient is to change. Someone can show up to a session with the best therapist in the world, but if he or she is there begrudgingly, the outcome is unlikely to be good. On the other hand, a patient who is highly motivated has a high chance of a successful outcome. What motivates you? Is there an image or person that comes to mind? If so, picture it every time you walk into a session."

52. We know that earlier is better for therapy, but how early should it start?

Dr. Carmichael: One thing that's emerging from studies of strokes, first in animals and now in humans, is that if you start too early, it may be harmful. There is a window immediately after a stroke during which intensive (or even normal) physical, occupational, or speech therapy may be harmful. The stroke destabilizes the brain; it takes a while to settle down after it occurs. After a while, the brain becomes stable again. If you get patients up and moving too vigorously while the brain is still unstable, that may be bad.

There are still a few things we don't know, such as how early is too early. Right now we know that about **three to five days after a stroke** is when we can really start to transition patients into more vigorous physical therapy, but we're not quite sure of the *exact* point. Another thing we're not quite sure of is how vigorous we can be. There's a lot of research being done at the moment to try to identify that information.

53. What is intensive therapy, and is it better than nonintensive therapy?

Dr. Carmichael: That's a very hot item of debate in the field. One thing we know is that physical, occupational, and speech therapy have a *dose effect*, just like a drug would. **The more therapy you get, the better you emerge** at the other end of the rehabilitation phase. What we don't know is exactly what that dose is or how intensive we can be.

There are studies indicating that there's a threshold below which therapy doesn't work. When everything is passively done for the patient, such as the arm being passively stretched or positioned, that appears not to be associated with much recovery. The patient has to engage the impaired function actively for at least a certain amount of time. We don't yet know how actively the patient has to engage it or for how long in order to see a recovery effect.

Right now, we actually have evidence that routine therapy, as long as it's delivered consistently and over time, is as good as intensive therapy. However, it's important to remember that the research settings that run these clinical trials are ideal situations. "Routine" therapy is what should happen in all places, but it often doesn't because patients fall through the cracks, or they have trouble getting to outpatient appointments, or other things like that happen. If a patient was to get six weeks of really good rehab therapy after discharge from the acute stroke service, right now that looks to be pretty good.

54. How is function different from impairment?

Dr. Gillen: *Functions* are the things we do in everyday life. Some functions are very mundane and we take them for granted, such as brushing our teeth, putting on our shoes, talking on the phone—everyday living. They can be simple things such as planning a meal or being on a bowling team or more complex things such as hosting Thanksgiving dinner or coaching your grandson's baseball team. It's a positive term; they're the things that you *can* do.

Impairment is a negative term. Impairments are the aftermath of a stroke that weaken our ability to function—things such as problems with balance, weak muscles, or difficulty with writing. An impairment has a negative effect on function.

Without a doubt, it's better to work on improving function rather than simply focusing on reducing impairments, especially after the first year. Some of the impairments won't get better, but we can still improve function by using adaptive techniques or different strategies. **So despite having impairments, people can still engage in different functional activities.** Improving function is the key for quality of life. It's also the key for insurance reimbursement.

◇◇◇

A stroke survivor asks, "If I focus too much on the adaptive strategies, will that prevent me from recovering the ability to do the task?"

Dr. Gillen: That's a valid concern. No therapist will ever give up on remediation. We'll often use what we call a *dual treatment plan*, where we're teaching people to do the task by **combining adaptive strategies and targeting the impairment.** Sometimes the strategies, or work-arounds, are a bridge to function. In the short term, we need to do things a different way until neurological, motor, or cognitive recovery occurs. Then we can systematically withdraw the strategies so the stroke survivor can do things more typically. So a strategy or tool might be a short-term way to solve a problem, and then in the long term people don't use it anymore. It's an "and" approach, rather than an "either/or" approach.

◇◇

55. What is mental practice and how does it help stroke survivors?

Dr. Page: Mental practice is something that has been around for decades in athletics. It's done by **mentally rehearsing something that you're physically doing.** The classic example is when you see Olympians mentally rehearsing a routine, dive, or whatever they're about to do. Then they physically do it. We know from decades of research that when people mentally and physically practice, their learning rate is faster, their skill acquisition is enhanced, and their outcomes are better.

About 15 years ago, we applied this tried-and-true concept to stroke rehab for the first time because we recognized that patients would do their physical practice and then go home or back to their hospital rooms and not have much to do. Now we know that when stroke survivors mentally rehearse the activities that they're doing in therapy, they get twice as much practice and, not surprisingly, their outcomes are better.

A great example of an activity to practice mentally is walking. I don't necessarily want my patients to go home and practice walking, because they could fall. Instead, I can give them the appropriate walking training while they're in the clinic and then provide them with an audio or video file to use at home. We know that when people listen to audio of being led through a walking sequence on various surfaces or observe a video of other people walking appropriately, it turns on the same parts of the brain and activates the muscles as if they're actually doing the activity themselves. Mental practice has some serious science behind it—it's not just fluffy stuff that athletes use. The bottom line is that when people go home and mentally practice walking, they're not physically practicing it, so the therapist doesn't have to worry about their safety, but they are getting some of the same repetitions in the muscles and in the brain as if they're actually doing it. That is enough to improve.

56. What should a stroke survivor look for in a therapist?

Dr. Page: There's no black-and-white answer. Some people will say, "Well, you need an experienced therapist," but my experience has been that sometimes the whippersnappers have new tricks that the experienced therapists don't know about. Therapists are trained differently; they're also trained at different times. It doesn't mean they're better or worse; it just means that they might have some different ideas about how to get at that impairment.

I would look for a therapist who doesn't just know about the exercises for your arm, leg, or speech and has a license and letters behind his or her name, but someone who actually **has a support team around them, is aware of the resources, and is up on what's going on in the field**. Someone who takes the time to go to conferences and read journals about stroke.

Dr. Holland: First of all, you want to work with someone who is as interested in you as he or she is in your impairments. Secondly, an ideal therapist is willing to work, not only with you, but also with your family and the other people whom you would like to have included. This is especially important for speech therapy since you don't communicate on your own. And finally, **a good therapist will be willing to work on what *you* want to work on**, rather than some set of assumptions of what you should be working on. One of my friends says, "Who would go to a hairdresser who says, 'I'm going to color your hair black,' without asking you if that's what you want?" So, a good therapist is one who basically says, "What can I do that will help you make the changes you want, be interesting for you, and involve the people who matter to you?"

"If you don't like your therapist, get another one. Over the years I have had many therapists. As in any profession, there are some good ones and some not so good ones. I didn't want to waste my time if I didn't think my therapist was good. And I worked harder if I liked my therapist and wanted to be there. Find someone who you work well with. It may not always be fun or enjoyable, but make sure you feel like you have someone who is on your side."
— *David*

A Tip from Dr. Mike

"A therapeutic relationship is a relationship, and you either click or you don't. It's important to find a professional you feel is a good fit for you. But don't discount people too soon, either. Sometimes a person we don't like at first becomes a good friend. Go into each session with a professional with an open mind. He or she may have a unique and valuable lesson to teach."

57. What does it mean when a doctor or therapist says a stroke survivor has "hit a plateau"?

Dr. Page: I actually hate the word *plateau,* and in my seminars to clinicians I tell them not to use it. *Plateau* means "flat." A plateau in stroke recovery implies that the amount of recovery a patient is exhibiting has flatlined a bit. What bothers me about that is that it implies that it's the patient's fault and that nothing can be done about it.

Therapists usually have to document your recovery. We have to document what happens and report it to the insurance company. If we can't continue to show that you're progressing toward your goals, then the insurance company won't pay for your care anymore or it will limit the number of visits. So it could be true that someone has stopped showing a measurable response to the current therapy goals, so the therapist had to discharge the person from therapy because the insurance company wouldn't pay anymore because of the lack of documented progress. Therapists need to explain this to families, then follow up by saying, "Here are some ways you can extend the quality care I've been providing your loved one in your home environment," and then provide more education and exercises.

58. What can a stroke survivor do when therapy has stalled out?

Dr. Page: Sometimes it's not a plateau of the patient; it's a plateau of the therapist. The therapist has done everything he or she knows, but it's not enough. You might have to go to a bigger town or a specialized center to get that really specialized, cutting-edge sort of care that will start to show results. Or just **switch therapists**. Find one with a new bag of tricks.

You can also get involved in a **research program** or clinical trial. People like me run research studies, and we're able to provide stroke survivors with things that usually aren't available in their communities, and sometimes aren't available anywhere else in the country or the world. We can jump-start their recoveries by providing those novel things. There are hundreds and hundreds of studies now suggesting that people might hit some sort of plateau in their movement or their recovery trajectory—whatever that might be—but they're able to jump-start it through the provision of a new therapy. If you want to get involved in research and be part of a study, go to clinicaltrials. gov to search for trials near your home. Clinical trials are a fantastic way for people to get cutting-edge care, and they don't depend on insurance.

Even if you can't get into a study, **academic medical centers** tend to have a lot of stuff going on. I work at a university and have to stay sharp because I have over 40 students who are asking me specific questions every day about different therapies and diagnoses. When I go treat, I'm often treating people with very challenging cases, people who have been turned away by other institutions. Those things keep up the skills of professionals working in these settings. In addition to that, my colleagues and I are doing research, so we have our hands on the pulse of what is going on in stroke rehabilitation. In this environment, I'm incentivized to do research, to provide cutting-edge clinical care, and to bring in new ways of thinking about therapy. You don't necessarily get that out in the community, unless it's a really special place.

Dr. Carmichael: The stroke survivor should **explore with a neurologist or a physiatrist** the things that he or she may have accidentally dropped off, or ways in which he or she has become static or less active. Unfortunately, we do slow down in recovery. The brain is uniquely plastic for a period of time after a stroke, and then that plasticity—that recovery potential—declines. We have to recognize that we're not going to have ongoing substantial recovery for a lifetime after a stroke, but if we're declining or if the recovery seems like it has plateaued, and there's a sense that it still could be improving, then it's worth talking to a health professional to identify what might be leading to that.

Setting SMART Goals

Therapists often set goals for you, but the most important goals are the ones you set for yourself. Goals should be SMART:

- Specific: the goal is clear and unambiguous.
- Measurable: the goal can be seen and measured in a concrete way.
- Attainable: the goal is realistic; it may be challenging, but it's not out of reach.
- Relevant: the goal is worthwhile.
- Time based: the goal has a specific target date.

Set a SMART goal for yourself now, and continue to set new SMART goals on a regular basis. This exercise helps you break down the journey into actionable steps, setting you up for success. If you can't find a way to measure a goal, record a video of yourself. Over time, you'll notice improvements in the quality of your movements or speech.

Here's an example of how to take an overwhelming thought and turn it into a SMART goal:

"I don't know if I'll ever walk again."
→ "I will walk two extra lengths of the parallel bars in physical therapy this week."

"My speech has to get so much better."
→ "I will call my daughter twice a week, and I will use my speech-therapy app for 30 minutes every day."

"I'm so overwhelmed, but my husband needs me."
→ "I will ask the neighbor to come over this weekend for a few hours to help so I can go out for coffee with a friend."

"We have so many bills to pay, and I don't know if I will ever go back to work. What are we going to do?"
→ "As I'm focusing on my recovery, my wife and I will cut our monthly expenses by $100 by the end of this month."

"Set realistic goals that are very small—and build on them. Don't set goals that are huge—it is disappointing. For example, one of my goals was to walk again. When I focused only on walking, it was disappointing. So I set smaller goals, like first being able to stand between the parallel bars in the rehab clinic. Then I built strength and movement slowly but surely. It takes time. Lots of time. Be patient. Focus on what you want to achieve today or this week." — David

59. What can stroke survivors do when their therapy ends?

Dr. Carmichael: Eventually, **life becomes therapy.** If somebody has a speech problem and is out and talking with people, that's a wonderful way to engage those neural circuits and get them going. I had a patient who was a bridge master, and he couldn't play bridge initially after his stroke. He started to go through quite a substantial decline, so we worked out a way for him to use online bridge programs. The minute he got back into his bridge group, his recovery took off because he was socially engaged and much more active. That's a good goal in the recovery period: getting patients back into their communities in ways in which they can engage and really accelerate the recovery process. If you're doing the things you love, you're going to be more motivated to do them.

Options When Therapy Ends from Megan

When you're discharged from therapy, it doesn't mean your recovery has come to an end. It simply means it's time to find a new way to keep that recovery going. When you're ready to start again, look into one or several of these options:

- **University clinics:** College campuses often have free or low-cost clinics used to train future health-care providers; there are excellent programs supervised by licensed professionals.

- **Research studies:** Go to clinicaltrials.gov to find stroke studies that are recruiting participants.

- **Check insurance renewal periods:** Sometimes coverage limits or caps reset each year, so you may be eligible for more therapy.

- **Get rereferred when you notice a change:** If something changes in your abilities, for better or for worse, you may be eligible for more therapy.

- **Join a stroke group:** Local stroke groups often have classes led by therapists or trained volunteers.

Meeting other stroke survivors provides support and shared experience to spark new ideas and solutions.

- **Home programs:** If you've fallen off the practice exercises last prescribed by your therapist, it's never too late to go back and renew your commitment to doing those home programs.

- **Technology:** There may be apps, videos, or games you can use at home for ongoing recovery. There are also online stroke groups on Facebook that provide support and ideas.

- **Private therapy:** Paying out of pocket for therapy may be an option, even if simply to get your home program updated or to get a series of consultations to see where you should be working next.

- **Teletherapy:** If you can't connect with a stroke recovery expert locally, look to see if one is available via teletherapy.

- **Get back into life:** Find a new hobby; join a new group; volunteer; learn a new sport, language, or instrument; plan a vacation; create a new craft; try a new recipe; write a blog—all of life can be therapeutic when you challenge yourself.

60. What can stroke survivors do when they feel hopeless and unmotivated to continue with their therapy?

Dr. Roth: First of all, there's an important distinction between hope and expectation. There's always hope. There's always possibility, there's always opportunity, and we always maintain hope. Having said that, it's also important to be realistic about what's expected. At some point, it's very helpful to have some acceptance of the current level of impairment and the expected long-term level of disability.

It's also valuable to begin thinking about satisfying other meaningful issues in a person's life. I've had a number of patients who've said to me, "You know, doc, this is the best thing that's happened to me." I say, "How is that possible?" They say it's taught them the value of their family and what is really important in life. Many of them aren't able to go to work, but they're able to interact with their children and do other things that really matter. The subtler things in their lives—the things that they never noticed before—become more prominent.

The Warrior's Ethos from Dr. Mike

On his last night in the hospital, David got a watch from his doctor with a soldier on it. It was a reminder for him to fight. Stroke survivors are indeed warriors. What follows is "The Warrior in Transition Mission Statement," which the US Army uses to remind their wounded warriors in transition—soldiers who have suffered a major injury, lost a limb, or are learning to walk again—of their mission. The mission is not over. It has simply changed. Even if they are unable to return to the battlefield because of a disability, they are still warriors. In fact, the bravery required for this mission of transition may be even greater than the threat of the battlefield.

The Warrior's Ethos
I will always place the mission first.
I will never accept defeat.
I will never quit.
I will never leave a fallen comrade.
I am a warrior in transition.
My job is to heal as I transition back to duty or continue serving the nation as a veteran in my community.
This is not a status, but a mission.
I will succeed in this mission because I AM A WARRIOR AND I AM ARMY STRONG.

Like the brave men and women who have served our country, stroke survivors and their loved ones may also find a mission statement empowering when it comes to recovery.

They too need to remember the incredible bravery this new mission requires. They too need to be reminded that their life's mission isn't gone even though it may have changed. Read this adapted ethos for stroke survivors and their loved ones. Fill in the last sentence with something that feels true for you.

The Stroke Warrior's Ethos
I will always place the recovery mission first.
I will never accept defeat.
I will never quit.
I will never leave a fallen survivor.
I am a Stroke Warrior in Transition.
My job is to heal or help my loved one heal.
My job is to heal as I transition back to my previous role or continue serving my community and family in a new way.
This is not a status, but a mission.
I will succeed in this mission because _____
_____.

•••••

Takeaway Points:

Maximize your time in therapy by learning exercises to do at home, having family members attend with you, and decreasing your time of not doing anything.

Therapy should be active, intensive, and plentiful. It should focus on improving function through a combination of remediating impairments and providing strategies to participate in activities despite those impairments.

Mental practice of therapy activities is a free, effective, and risk-free way to improve faster.

Look for a therapist who is part of a stroke team, who keeps up on the latest in stroke recovery, and who cares about you and what you want.

Sometimes a stroke survivor will stop making progress on a goal, hitting a plateau. It could be that the goal isn't right, a different approach is called for, or the therapist should be replaced. Look to join a research program or get therapy at an academic medical center. Go back to your neurologist or physiatrist to see if there's anything they can recommend.

When therapy ends, think of the ways that you can make your life part of your therapy. There may be stroke groups, university clinics, or other therapy options available. Carry on with your home exercises, and use technology to continue your recovery.

Use your family members and friends to get out into the community, and let them challenge you. There is always hope, so don't give up! Focus on what matters to you.

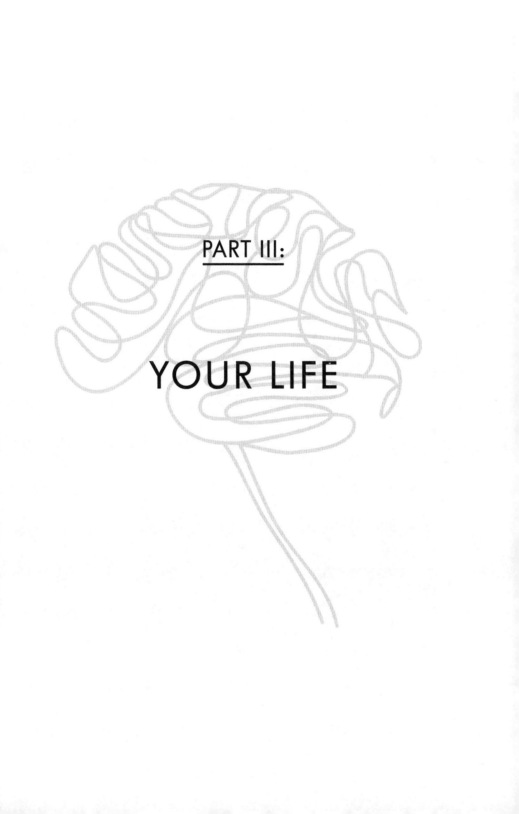

PART III:

YOUR LIFE

CHAPTER 9

RECOVERING YOUR HEALTH

Your stroke may have been caused by a variety of health problems, but it puts you at risk for even more. If your mobility is impaired, it will be more difficult to exercise. If your income is reduced, it may be harder to eat right or get the medical care you need. It's important now more than ever to make sure you're doing everything you can to optimize your health, both to improve your recovery and to prevent further complications. We asked the experts about the optimal nutrition, exercise, and rest for stroke survivors' overall health.

61. What should stroke survivors do to improve their health after a stroke?

Dr. Hinkle: The things that are important for all of us, such as diet, exercise, and good sleep, become even more important for a great recovery after a stroke. Actually, this applies to both the stroke survivor and the caregiver. Both should try to be in optimal health in order to get back to as many of their normal activities as possible. **Try to eat three nutritious meals a day, sleep eight hours every night, and get some exercise.**

Dr. Ploughman: We know that someone who has had a stroke is at high risk of having another one, so you want to do everything possible to improve your lifestyle in order to reduce your stroke risk. You can improve your diet by reducing saturated fat, eating lots of fruits and vegetables, and reducing salt. Definitely increase your physical activity. Try to hit a target of at least 30 minutes of moderate exercise three times a week—at an intensity where you feel tired. And absolutely **stop smoking** as soon as you can.

"Have a good relationship with your doctor, and allow time to discuss issues. If you need help, bring a caregiver. Practice what you want to say beforehand, or write your thoughts down. Ask the doctor to write down key words so you can go home and research more. Become your own advocate." — David

A Tip from Dr. Mike

"A stroke survivor's loved one often takes on the advocate role immediately after a stroke. As a stroke survivor regains function, it's important for loved ones to hand as much responsibility as possible back to the survivor. This helps a family move from a state of enabling the survivor to being in a passive recovery role to empowering the survivor to take charge of his or her own recovery. This sense of power and mastery is something we all need in our lives. It also is a powerful antidote to prevent depression."

62. What is the best diet for a stroke survivor in recovery?

Dr. Roth: When patients first come to me in inpatient rehab, I tell them that one of the two most important things to remember is nutrition. (The other is sleep.) We emphasize the need for **protein intake**. Stroke survivors are using up a lot of energy, and they're trying to build up muscle. For immediate energy, they need some kind of carbohydrates. But basically after any kind of brain injury, there's a sizable amount of protein loss, so we urge people to eat protein. There's good research on how protein levels improve outcomes after stroke, so it's quite important.

Typically we recommend one gram of protein per kilogram (2.2 pounds) of weight per day. For people who have other medical problems, which many people do following stroke, we'll go up 1.2 or 1.5 grams per kilogram. I prefer to have people get their protein by eating high-protein foods rather than by using supplements or powders. I tell them to eat lean meat, fish, turkey, peanut butter, or eggs.

Many stroke survivors have problems with constipation or bowel function, so I always recommend **fruits and vegetables** for the fiber and other nutrients too. The problem is that a lot of people are eating junk food, which may be what led them to have a stroke in the first place, so trying to change those habits into better food choices is a big challenge.

Dr. Chiu: Diet is so important. Patients think, "Oh well, here's my doctor once again telling me how important it is to eat right and to exercise," but these are critical. We talk about stroke being preventable, but that doesn't mean that it's going to be easy. We know the tools. Every physician tells every patient to eat right, no matter what the condition is. It goes double for preventing another stroke.

Reducing sodium is essential—you have to cut your salt intake from processed and prepared food. **Reducing carbs** and eating a Mediterranean diet is also highly recommended. It can help with the control of diabetes and *metabolic syndrome* (high blood pressure, blood sugar, cholesterol, and body weight). The Mediterranean diet has data supporting that it can improve heart health and reduce the risk of vascular disease, including stroke. For people who aren't familiar with it, the **Mediterranean diet** is a diet high in fresh fruits, vegetables, fish, whole grains, and olive oil.

The Modified Mediterranean Diet from Dr. Mike

Many of the principles in my book *The Brain Fog Fix* are especially important for stroke survivors. Remember: stroke is the second leading cause of dementia, so all the strategies that have been linked to dementia prevention are vital if you've had a stroke. For overall brain health, I recommend a modified Mediterranean diet. It's "modified" because it is very low in processed carbohydrates, including flour and sugar; it is high in beans, vegetables, whole fruits, omega-3 superfoods like wild salmon, and healthy fats like olive oil; and it's low in the saturated fats you find in American pepperoni pizza and cheese. Most Americans think of pasta and pizza when they think of Italy, but the pepperoni pizza and spaghetti and meatballs Americans eat have no place in this type of diet.

Spiking your blood sugar with too many processed carbohydrates and too much soda, bread, pasta, flour, sugar, and high-fructose corn syrup can interfere with the brain's ability to rewire. Factory-farmed animal products have high levels of omega-6s that lead to inflammation in the body and brain. You need *some* carbohydrates, but most people around the world eat far too many processed carbohydrates. And, research shows a low-carbohydrate diet may protect the brain. A clinical trial is now under way to examine the effect of a low-carbohydrate diet on poststroke recovery in survivors.

In addition to this clinical trial, a number of recent studies have shed light on how a modified Mediterranean diet may help stroke survivors. In 2015, UCLA research demonstrated that high-sugar diets, specifically diets that contained large amounts of processed fructose in the form of high-fructose corn syrup, interfered with the brain's ability to heal from traumatic injury. While a stroke is not a traumatic brain injury, it is similar in that both conditions require the brain to grow new cells and rewire for optimal recovery. The research team found the sweetener "interfered with the ability of neurons to communicate with each other, rewire connections after injury, record memories, and produce enough energy to fuel basic functions." It prevented neuroplasticity—the birth of new brain cells—that is critical to a stroke survivor's brain rewiring.

Another study, which was published in *The New England Journal of Medicine*, found that 30 percent of strokes, heart attacks, and deaths from heart disease can be prevented by following a Mediterranean diet. The dietary changes in the study included eating **extra-virgin olive oil and/or nuts daily, fish three or more times a week, beans three or more times a week, white meat instead of red meat, at least three daily servings of fruits, and two daily servings of vegetables.**

A study published in *Frontiers in Nutrition* found subjects following a Mediterranean diet showed improvements in language, attention, and memory. And a groundbreaking 2016 study found that people who followed a Mediterranean diet had larger brains: the frontal, parietal, and occipital lobes were actually thicker. Of the foods in the Mediterranean diet, **fish** and **beans** were found to be especially associated with thicker brain structures. In this same study, the subjects who consumed large amounts of carbohydrates and sugar had smaller brains, as those same lobes were thinner. For stroke survivors, retaining remaining brain cells and growing new ones through neuroplasticity is vital.

Vegetables and whole fruits are a vital part of a modified Mediterranean diet as well. Eating at least five servings daily has been shown to reduce stroke risk significantly. In *The Brain Fog Fix* I recommend a whopping seven servings of vegetables and whole fruits a day, as this is how many servings the healthiest and happiest people around the world reported eating. Cruciferous vegetables like broccoli, kale, cauliflower, and brussels sprouts may be especially helpful in reducing stroke risk, but you should also talk to your doctor if you are taking the blood thinner Coumadin, since vitamin K in these vegetables can interfere with this medication. Talk to you doctor to see if there are any dietary restrictions with any of the medications you are taking.

You've probably heard of omega-3s, which are found in seafood like wild salmon. Of the three types of omega-3s, docosahexaenoic acid (DHA) is probably the most beneficial to stroke survivors. DHA helps to maintain healthy cognition, prevents dementia, and acts as a building block for the brain.

Pregnant mothers need DHA to support their infants' brain development, and stroke survivors need DHA to promote neurogenesis and the rewiring of their brain. The best source of DHA is seafood. Here is a list of seafood-based omega-3 superfoods that are high in DHA omega-3 and also low in toxins like mercury: albacore tuna (troll or pole caught), farmed arctic char, farmed barramundi, farmed coho salmon, wild Dungeness crab, wild longfin squid, farmed mussels, farmed oysters, wild sardines, shrimp, farmed rainbow trout, wild salmon, and wild prawns. According to the most recent research, eating a serving of one of these at least three times a week can support brain health and recovery. One of the cheapest and easiest ways to do this is to find wild salmon in vacuum-sealed packs next to the tuna in the grocery store. Farmed rainbow trout is another favorite of mine, as it's mild and inexpensive. While they won't provide as much DHA as seafood, plant-based sources such as walnuts, chia seeds, and flaxseed can provide vegetarians with some DHA.

Here is a summary of the simple changes you can make in your diet to help heal your broken brain:

- The best protein foods for brain health are seafood and beans. Eat them regularly. When eating seafood, favor the varieties in the list above. These are high in DHA omega-3s and low in toxins like mercury.

- Eat less meat in general. When you do eat meat, favor grilled chicken over red meat. When you eat animal products, favor organic, grass-fed, or pastured varieties over conventional varieties. This is true for dairy products and eggs as well. These types of animal products have more anti-inflammatory omega-3s and fewer pro-inflammatory omega-6s compared to conventional varieties of meat, dairy, and eggs.

- Olive oil is the best oil to use for overall brain health. Use extra-virgin olive oil for dressings and salads. Extra-virgin is not stable at high temperatures, however, so use light or plain olive oil for cooking. Reduce or eliminate industrial vegetable oils (such as corn oil and soybean oil) that are found in most processed foods.

- Eat more nuts. Favor any kind of nut over peanuts, since peanuts are not a true tree nut like walnuts, almonds, cashews, and pistachios. Look for plain nuts rather than nuts cooked in oil, as the oils tend to be high in pro-inflammatory omega-6s.

- Reduce or eliminate flour, sugar, and artificial sweeteners. If you need a sweetener, choose stevia. Favor healthy grains like quinoa, barley, sprouted grains, and brown rice. Get carbohydrates from whole fruits and beans. Reduce your carbohydrate intake by substituting cauliflower or broccoli for pasta. Make cauliflower rice or buy frozen varieties. Use a vegetable peeler to make zucchini noodles, or use spaghetti squash in lieu of noodles. When you eat a sandwich, order it wrapped in lettuce instead of bread, eat just one of the pieces of bread, or, if you're eating somewhere that serves sandwiches on big rolls, ask for your bread to be shelled out (the inner bread pulled away and discarded, which reduces the amount of flour you'll consume). If you're eating pizza, favor thin crust over thicker crust to reduce the carbohydrate content.

- Aim for five to seven whole fruits and vegetables a day. Again, check with your doctor for any interactions with prescription medication—especially if you're taking Coumadin, since vitamin K can interfere with this drug.

63. Are there any vitamins or supplements stroke survivors should take?

Dr. Chiu: There's not a lot of evidence suggesting that stroke survivors should be taking specific vitamins or supplements, but a general one-a-day multivitamin that contains **B vitamins including folic acid** may very well be beneficial. There is now a fairly strong and established link between folic acid deficiency and an increased risk of stroke.

I don't recommend any of the other supplements marketed for brain health. We don't always know what is contained in those supplements, and it's very hard for medical professionals to recommend things when we don't know what's in them or what complications they might create.

Dr. Carmichael: Most of the "natural" supplements have never really been tested, so there's **no clinical evidence to support them.** They fall into this big "alternative medicine" bin. Patients pay out of pocket, and the supplements can be quite expensive. I don't routinely recommend them, especially if they're pushed by an herbal medicine company that deliberately tries to keep them out of the medical realm. Herbal medicines are not regulated by the FDA (Food and Drug Administration), so they don't have to be tested for the claims made by the manufacturers, which can make them quite profitable for those companies. I usually don't recommend any of those to my patients since they're not tested.

If you're considering taking supplements, talk to your doctor before you do. Some are known to be harmful. There are bad mixtures of herbal and alternative medicines that can have effects on the liver, or other **dangerous side effects**, so these supplements should be avoided. As for the other ones, I simply tell my patients that there's no evidence that they work and that they can be expensive, so **don't put yourself at financial risk** by pursuing them.

"One of my concerns is bogus claims. Sometimes companies claim 'quick fixes,' but I haven't seen any. I am wary of products and programs that sell false hope. Stroke survivors are a

vulnerable population—we want a quick fix and we need hope. I'd advise people to be very cautious. There are medications, foods, and therapies that help recovery, but there is probably no 'miracle' cure. You and your hard work will become the greatest miracle." — David

A Tip from Dr. Mike

"No matter the problem, people tend to use polarized, black-or-white thinking when it comes to healing. One therapy didn't work immediately, so they abandon it completely. The next week, they're onto some other treatment that is going to be the 'cure-all.' In most cases, it's more gray area and less black or white. For most survivors, a combination of different strategies, therapies, medications, and lifestyle choices will collectively optimize their personal recovery journey."

64. Is it safe to drink caffeine or alcohol after having a stroke?

Dr. Chiu: Moderate caffeine intake has not been shown to be a risk factor for stroke. So for those patients who have had a stroke and want to have a cup or two of coffee or tea, it's not a problem.

Assuming that there are no other medical issues that would impact the safety of drinking alcohol, moderate alcohol intake is not a stroke risk factor either. "Moderate" means **a maximum of one to two drinks a day**. On the other hand, excessive alcohol consumption does increase the risk of stroke. Talk to your doctor first to make sure alcohol consumption is safe for you with the medications you're taking.

◇◇

A stroke survivor says, "I have difficulty swallowing. Why is this, and what can I do about it?"

Dr. Hinckley: Difficulty swallowing is known as *dysphagia*, and it's very common immediately after a stroke. Some swallowing problems have to do with problems in the mouth, and some have to do with problems in the throat or farther down. Because there are different types and causes of dysphagia, there are different ways to manage them. The best thing is to be properly evaluated by a speech-language pathologist. You may get suggestions about the type and texture of food that is safest or easiest to swallow. Sometimes there are certain positions or exercises that can help. All of these recommendations are specific to the nature of the problem, so the **first step is to get evaluated.** It's very important to make sure you are swallowing safely to prevent getting pneumonia and to keep nourished and hydrated.

◇◇

65. How much exercise should a stroke survivor get?

Dr. Ploughman: It depends on the type of exercise. If we're talking about task-specific training—things like reaching tasks or placing your leg in the right position to walk again—you'll probably need to do thousands of repetitions of those tasks in order for the brain to rewire and for you to regain the ability to do those tasks again.

In terms of strengthening and aerobic fitness, we know you need to do that **two or three times a week at moderate intensity** to see any real functional gain. How much is enough depends on the type of exercise and what you want to improve.

66. Is it safe for stroke survivors to go back to the gym after a stroke, or do they need special exercise equipment or supervision?

Dr. Ploughman: Going back to the gym is a good idea and a smart thing to do. **Check with your family doctor first**, though, because your stroke may have been related to a problem with your heart, high blood pressure, or something that can cause problems with exercise. Also, when you use heavy weights, you tend to hold your breath, and that can increase your blood pressure. So you need to know from your family doctor if your blood pressure or atrial fibrillation is being controlled well enough for you to exercise.

If you don't have any problems with your heart or high blood pressure, you can probably go to the gym. The challenge is that in the real world, gyms are made for people who don't have any disability. Getting on and off the machines may not be easy for you. It's good practice to get the help of a physical therapist for your first few visits. If you don't have a physical therapist around, you can probably talk to a personal trainer or a kinesiologist who has a good background in helping people with stroke about how best to start exercising again.

67. How helpful are treatments like yoga, acupuncture, and massage?

Dr. Carmichael: Yoga can have a positive role in recovery. It's a way to be physically active and use the postures to stretch and enhance flexibility. It doesn't replace structured use of the impaired function, but I encourage patients to get out and be physical. So if yoga is their thing, that's great.

Acupuncture has a role for chronic pain. However, even in well-established acupuncture clinics, only about 30 percent of patients will experience the pain-relief benefit. It has less of a role with strokes since there's no evidence that acupuncture works to promote brain plasticity or recovery in stroke, and it can be expensive.

Massage is a passive treatment. The patient isn't actively engaging in the recovery process, but it can have benefits in terms of reducing anxiety and pain. However, if it takes away from the time the patient has to devote to being active and pursuing active recovery, then it's not good.

68. What about hyperbaric oxygen treatment?

Dr. Carmichael: Hyperbaric oxygen therapy (HBOT) is a treatment that hyperoxygenates the blood by putting a person in a pressurized chamber. HBOT is approved for only a few things in the United States, including diabetic ulcers on the legs and the bends (nitrogen damage from rapidly surfacing when deepwater diving), but it **hasn't been approved for stroke**. In the early stages of stroke, a clot is blocking a blood vessel. However, after the first three days, the blood is flowing normally again, so there isn't a problem of low oxygen in the brain.

The idea that putting somebody in a hyperbaric oxygen chamber will enhance recovery is just **not scientifically supported**. The person doesn't have an oxygen deficit anymore. The problem is that everybody feels a little boost when the blood is hyperoxygenated, so there's a strong placebo effect, but it isn't sustained. There is no actual mechanism of enhanced repair in the brain or enhanced recovery. Unfortunately, there are a lot of stroke survivors suffering without proven treatments, so there is a big market for alternative treatments. Entrepreneurs are more than happy to provide hope and charge you quite a bit to go into their expensive machine without any guarantee of results.

69. How does sleep impact recovery, and how important is sleep for somebody who has had a stroke?

Dr. Roth: So much of stroke recovery emphasizes the importance of the individual's energy and effort, both of which require the person to be well rested. The stroke survivor has to have had **sufficient sleep to be able to put the effort into recovery**. Exhaustion is a common problem, and rehabilitation, if it's done right, can be very tiring. Sometimes people may actually have a somewhat easier time sleeping because they're working so hard during the day.

Unfortunately, there are many people who don't do a whole lot following their stroke, and many of them will have difficulty sleeping. Some people will take naps during the day, which interferes with sleeping at night more than most people realize. And some people have bad sleep habits—for example, drinking too much caffeine, watching TV, or doing something that's too stimulating before bedtime. They need to **change these habits** or behaviors to improve their sleep.

Doctors also can prescribe certain medications to help with sleep. I try to use natural medications whenever possible, because they have fewer side effects. We can use *melatonin* if someone is having trouble sleeping. It's sold in health food stores and pharmacies, and it's a natural hormone that exists in the body and helps many people sleep.

70. What can stroke survivors do if they feel fatigued all the time?

Dr. Roth: Fatigue, or *neurofatigue,* is a very common problem, and it's one that's receiving a tremendous amount of scientific investigation right now. It's very hard to measure fatigue or to conduct research studies on it because it's so subjective.

Quite honestly, the full cause of neurofatigue is not fully understood. I suspect it's partly that the brain is being asked to do a lot of things, but with part of the brain being injured, it doesn't have quite as much to work with. So the brain tissue that's remaining has to work that much harder, and it becomes exhausting. It's similar to what happens to the muscles in the body that start to compensate for the weaker muscles—they get overused. There are other theories on why it happens, like metabolic or *endocrine* changes—changes in hormone levels. It's a very important problem because of how pervasive and persistent it is in stroke and brain injury survivors. I have patients who have recovered fully or almost fully from their strokes and say their main remaining symptom is fatigue.

There aren't simple answers. Typically I will say, "**The best thing to do is to balance rest and exercise.**" Because they're fatigued, some people will just rest and spend their day being vegetative—watching

TV, sitting in a chair all day, taking a lot of naps, not doing too much. That's the wrong approach.

Having said that, I absolutely believe that working too hard will make the fatigue and other symptoms worse. In fact, there are two sets of symptoms that people have. One is that they feel pooped more frequently and earlier. And the other is that their performance gets worse when they get fatigued. So not only do they get tired out, but also when they're tired, they tend to walk a bit worse, their balance isn't as good, they're at greater risk for falls, they may talk with more slurred speech, and their arms may be weaker. Physical changes happen because they're fatigued.

What I adamantly tell people is "**We want you to work hard to the point of fatigue, but not through fatigue.**" The same with working *to* pain but not *through* pain. They have to be the judge of it, because nobody else can know when they're at that point. I don't say to them, "Work this number of hours," or "Walk that distance." I say, "Work as much as you can or walk as far as you can, but stop before you get fatigued. Don't push through it." Which is different from a lot of what we tell them in other things that we do, where we're pushing people beyond what they think is their limit.

Dr. Holland: It's very important for people in rehab to **let others know** when they are tired, when their energy is really low. It doesn't do any good for the quality of your rehabilitative experience if you try to do your therapy when you are very tired. Make sure that the staff understands the level of your energy and tries to work within it. That's an important concept throughout recovery. People with a variety of neurological problems tend to be fatigued and easily drained, and the therapists don't always remember that.

> *"I get tired a lot. The brain needs rest. They call this neurofatigue, and most of the stroke survivors I know have it. We need more sleep. And we tire easily when we use our brains. Before, I tired out easily when I used my muscles. But now at times it is tiring to use my brain too much as well. Make sure you are getting good sleep. Rest when you need it. But also make sure you are work-*

ing hard for your recovery. This includes staying active, staying connected, and exercising. As they say, use it or lose it." — David

A Tip from Dr. Mike

"Whole person-centered treatment is essential in recovery. Your physical health, psychological well-being, social life, and spirituality are all elements that must be addressed. Here's one example of how these aspects interact. Medications can affect sleep, and sleep can affect energy levels. Having higher levels of energy makes you more likely to connect with friends or work harder in therapy. Your beliefs or spiritual practices—through prayer, meditation, or nature—can help you find serenity in your journey. Make sure you aren't neglecting any of these needs, because each one is a piece of your healing process."

Dr. Chiu: If you're feeling tired all the time, first you'll want to make sure there isn't a medical condition aside from the stroke that's leading to the fatigue, like an infection or *anemia* (low count of red blood cells). Once you rule out other causes, ask why the stroke is leading to this feeling of being tired and fatigued. Part of it could be that it just takes greater effort for you to do things that you used to do without much effort. If you have trouble walking, getting from point A to point B now may take 10 times as long and 10 times as much effort. Also, about a third of people have *mood disorders* after a stroke; they have conditions like depression that can cause a feeling of being tired or fatigued.

Then there is also something called *obstructive sleep apnea*, a condition where you have pauses in your breathing during sleep. The hallmark of obstructive sleep apnea is being tired because you're not getting good oxygenation at night. You may be observed to snore, and you don't feel refreshed after a night's sleep because you're not getting enough oxygen to the brain. Sleep apnea can be both a cause and a result of stroke. The good news is that sleep apnea is a readily diagnosable and treatable condition, so it's worthwhile to get a screening for it if you have excessive daytime sleepiness after a stroke.

71. Is it safe for a stroke survivor to be sexually active again? Are there other issues for intimacy after a stroke that people should consider?

Dr. Chiu: Physical activity after a stroke is highly encouraged, particularly moderate aerobic physical activity, and I put sexual activity in that category. The last thing you want to do is become sedentary, become a couch potato.

There are other issues that can affect intimacy after a stroke. Mood problems, which are unfortunately quite prevalent, can affect feelings of intimacy and sometimes have an effect on performance or confidence. But in terms of the safety, for those who have the desire, it's to be highly encouraged.

Dr. Gillen: Many times sexual function is not discussed after a stroke. It might be because the therapist isn't comfortable with the topic, or because he or she makes an incorrect assumption that older adults don't have a sex life. That should never be the case. Sexual relations have to be considered as part of a partnership and as an activity of daily living.

Many times the sexual relationship stops because the partner is afraid of hurting the stroke survivor. Or they both might think it could cause another stroke, which is unfounded. Also, positions that were preferred before might be difficult or impossible to assume after a stroke.

Therapists can help you work through these issues in terms of choosing activities that partners can do together to have a relationship and that fulfill intimacy needs. The problem is that when we go from partner to caregiver, that's a whole switch in relationship dynamics. Sex and intimacy are part of our lives, and couples need to find a balance between caregiving and having a relationship.

◇◇◇

A stroke survivor asks, "Can I still have children after a stroke?"

Dr. Roth: Yes, a woman can still have children after a stroke. There is no impact of the stroke on fertility, on the ability to carry a baby, or on pregnancy, labor, or delivery. It may be a little more uncomfortable and difficult to carry the baby because the mechanics of movement change so much when the uterus is enlarged. And sometimes the person may have a very difficult time finding a comfortable position, but it's not a complication. I've seen many women who've had babies after having a stroke and they do fine. Talk to your doctor about your personal risk factors.

◇◇◇

• • • • •

TAKEAWAY POINTS:

Improving your diet, exercise, and sleep are the most important things you can do for your health after a stroke.

A low-sodium, low-carbohydrate diet that is also low in saturated fats is the healthiest. The Mediterranean diet—one high in fish, beans, fruits, vegetables, whole grains, lean meats, and olive oil—may be best.

There is no evidence to support the claim that taking any natural or vitamin supplements helps improve brain health. The exception to this is B-complex vitamins, including folic acid. Talk to your doctor before starting any new supplement as it may interact with your medications. It's important to exercise after a stroke. Before returning to the gym to exercise, talk to your doctor to make sure that your risk factors are under control. If you have mobility problems, enlist the help of a physical therapist or other exercise specialist.

Getting good sleep is very important. Don't eat or drink caffeine too close to bedtime, don't take naps if you have trouble sleeping at night, and stop taking part in stimulating activities and watching screens late at night. If you're having trouble sleeping, try melatonin before choosing regular sleeping pills.

Fatigue is one of the most bothersome and long-lasting problems for stroke survivors. Try to balance your rest and effort, and don't push through the fatigue. Talk to your doctor about your fatigue as there may be a treatable cause that is unrelated to your stroke.

Sexuality after a stroke is not something that should be ignored. Ask for advice on when it's safe to resume sexual activity and ways to modify your activities. The emotional and relationship components of sexuality are likely to be far more complicated than the physical aspects.

CHAPTER 10

RECOVERING YOUR LIFE

After a stroke, it can feel like your life has ended, even though you're still alive. That's because a stroke doesn't affect just your body and mind—it can also take away your independence, career, and hobbies. You'll need to figure out where you can live and what you can do in this new poststroke life. You may need to find new activities that give you purpose and bring you joy to make you feel truly alive again. To help us understand the process, we've brought in Dr. Janice Elich Monroe, the chair of the Department of Recreation and Leisure Studies at Ithaca College in New York and the clinical supervisor at the Center for Life Skills, a program serving stroke survivors. We also offer you the expertise of Dr. Amanda Woodward, a social worker, associate professor, and researcher at Michigan State University. Sarah Thompson, a music therapist specializing in stroke, adds valuable insights into how music therapy can enhance recovery too.

72. Many stroke survivors don't want to go home until they're fully recovered. What would you say to someone who doesn't feel he or she is ready to face regular life again?

Dr. Hinkle: A lot of people are probably ready to go home before the rehab team thinks they're ready. Recovery from a stroke takes a long time—6 months, 18 months, or longer. Home is usually the best place to make the most optimal recovery. It makes people nervous, but ultimately they're going to make their best recovery when they're in their normal, familiar environment doing everyday things for themselves. **Home is probably the best thing** for them.

The other part of this transition is that stroke survivors have to get used to their *new normal*. Life may never be the same as they knew it before the stroke. And that's okay. Every person who deals with this can find some part of his or her new life that is rewarding and fulfilling.

"It took a long time for me to realize my new potential and focus on the positive things—what I can do, not what I cannot do. I may not be able to be a doctor like I wanted, but I can still help people. I started a nonprofit organization to connect people with aphasia. It helps me focus on my abilities. But you don't have to start a nonprofit like I did to stay focused on your abilities. What are the things that help you stay positive? How do you focus on what you can do?" — David

A Tip from Dr. Mike

"Reflect on the Serenity Prayer—either as a prayer or a message that will help you to find acceptance and focus on your abilities: **God (or highest, wisest self), grant me the serenity to accept the things I cannot change, courage to change the things I can, and wisdom to know the difference.** What do *you* have the power to change in your life today?"

73. How can stroke survivors begin to regain their independence?

Dr. Monroe: It's all about focusing on what you can do, versus what you can't. It's also really important to be patient with yourself, and to be patient with other people, while recognizing there will be mistakes.

It's okay to make mistakes. A lot of times we are so afraid to say or do the wrong thing that we end up saying or doing nothing at all.

It's so important to remember what you can still do and build on that. Try to be yourself. Don't define yourself by your disability. Let your friends know that it's a priority for you to be the person that you are. You know that you've changed, but you're still the same person underneath with different abilities.

Remember too that all of us have some areas where we're dependent. I'm considered able-bodied, but I can't cut my own hair, so I depend on other people to do that for me. That dependency is accentuated a lot more if you have a disability, but don't forget that even before your stroke, you probably couldn't do everything for yourself or perfectly. So **be patient with yourself**, and recognize that you're not going to be able to do everything, because nobody can.

74. How can stroke survivors safely and successfully reenter their communities?

Dr. Monroe: This is one of the scariest parts for stroke survivors, not only because of their impaired ability to get around, but also because of the risk of being faced with people who may not be very considerate of their impairments. If your balance is not good and you're in a crowded place, people moving quickly might knock you over. So that's really scary, right? You don't want to fall and hurt yourself. It's important to start out in familiar environments that don't have a lot of obstacles, and **practice, practice, practice.** Find a place that you used to go to that you'd like to revisit, and go with someone who can be there for you if you need assistance but who knows that you want to do it on your own.

Being familiar with alternative modes of transportation and ways to get yourself around can really help with independence. Take a bus or a cab to the place first with somebody that you trust, and then do it on your own. Have somebody around that you can call to let him or her know when you get there, or if you need help. You don't need to jump back into the world all at once. You need to learn something, practice it, learn something new, practice it, get good at it, and continue on. Baby steps.

Author's note: Loving caregivers want to keep stroke survivors safe and protect them from harm. However, we all take risks in our lives, and those of us without disabilities get to determine what level of risk is acceptable. Taking risks, getting outside our comfort zones, and making mistakes are how we learn and improve. Overprotection can impede recovery by eliminating those valuable learning opportunities and making the survivor feel powerless. Try to find a balance between protection and self-determination to restore the "dignity of risk" in your stroke survivor.

◇◇

A stroke survivor asks, "How can I plan for the future when I don't know how far my recovery will go?"

Dr. Woodward: It's hard to think about the future, let alone make long-term plans, when you're trying to learn how to walk again. It's not a onetime conversation. Planning for the future is part of the recovery process.

Perhaps your immediate focus for recovery is learning to walk again, but learning to walk again to what end? Is your goal to go back to work? Maybe you want to use this as an opportunity to do a different kind of work, or maybe it's time to retire. Take the opportunity to **look at your future** in a different way.

Maybe your goal is to get back to exactly where you were and the life that you had before, but maybe it's something different. Finding some time to think about the future is integral to the overall recovery process and helpful for staying motivated and having goals to work toward.

Obviously, the future is going to look different for people of different ages and at different stages in their careers. Rehab professionals and social workers can help you plan for that future and help you understand what the options are. Talking to other stroke survivors who have been in your shoes, as well as to professionals, can help you understand the resources available to lay out different options for you.

◇◇

75. How can stroke survivors manage financial stress while they're recovering?

Dr. Woodward: This is a question that people often put off thinking about, but as soon as it's feasible, you need to start thinking about finances. Even though it's hard, dealing with it **sooner rather than later** will actually help alleviate some of the stress in the long term. Create a budget and prioritize your expenses. You need to keep paying your health insurance premiums. Talk with your landlord or your lender early on if you think you're going to have issues with paying. Let him or her know what has happened, and see if he or she can help you figure out options.

One of the first things a social worker will do is assess all of your current and anticipated needs in order to help you figure out what has to be addressed and to connect you with available resources. There are local and federal housing-assistance programs and other programs that can help you pay utilities or get food. You can call 211 just like 911 to get help with figuring out what resources are available in your community. There is also a website (www.211.org) where you can enter your zip code to find local resources and help you navigate the maze of options.

76. What percentage of stroke survivors return to work?

Dr. Roth: The figures are terrible, frankly. It's estimated that about one third of people will go back to work following a stroke. Even in programs that focus heavily on pushing people to get back to work, where all the therapy is directed toward work issues, that number maybe gets pushed as high as 50 percent.

In rehabilitation we have made lots of progress with helping people learn how to walk, use their arms, take care of themselves, and to a lesser extent get back into the community. But we have not done as much as we should have with helping stroke survivors return to work.

Work can be part of recovery. Work can be therapy in a lot of ways. If you're getting up and going to work, whether it's a part-time job or a full-time job, you're being forced to use your brain on a consistent basis and be more physically active. My observation is that people who are back at work are less likely to get medical illnesses, spend less time in the hospital, and have fewer other problems. They seem to be less depressed too, probably because they feel like they're contributing more. There are lots of good, objective medical reasons to go back to work, in addition to it being good to get back to your normal life and earn a paycheck.

77. What are the barriers to returning to work?

Dr. Roth: There are many reasons why stroke survivors have difficulty returning to work. One reason is discrimination and prejudice on the part of employers. Another is the lack of accessibility—physical accessibility as well as breaking down attitudinal barriers of employers. A more hidden reason is that medical professionals and communities at large do not have enough of an expectation that stroke survivors can and should be working.

I was part of a team researching employment for people with strokes. To help people get back to work, we started focusing on the employers. We worked directly with the companies to get them thinking about what modifications for people with strokes may be needed, required by law, and reasonable. We got a lot of interest from high-level executives in companies, which we thought was a great thing. However, it turns out that what matters most is not what the corporate philosophy is, but what the immediate supervisors and co-workers think—what their attitudes are. If they're prejudiced, bitter, or resentful in any way, then there's a problem. Of course, most clinicians aren't really thinking about that in the rehab process, but that ends up driving much of the success for people returning to work. There are laws that prohibit this kind of discrimination, so you can fight it, but you have to recognize when that's the problem.

78. If a stroke survivor can't return to work, what can he or she do?

Dr. Monroe: In our society we are defined by what we do for work. When you don't work, it's really important to be able to replace that identity with something else. You need to **find meaningful activity that gives you purpose.** If a stroke survivor is not working, he or she may have more free time, at least after all the doctor appointments are over. To gain back your confidence, it's important to find things to do that keep you engaged physically, mentally, cognitively, and socially. These may be activities that enable you to get back into the workplace, if that is a goal, or they may just be activities that are meaningful, provide you with purpose, and give you a new sense of identity.

Dr. Carmichael: A great example of a man who's very active in stroke recovery is Reams Freedman in Southern California. He suffered a stroke and now runs the Stroke Association of Southern California, a volunteer stroke-survivor network. I'm sure if you had sat him down 20 years ago and asked if he was going to be doing this sort of thing, he would have said "No way," but he really took charge and has been integral in a lot of people's recoveries and lives. So there are certainly opportunities that open up to patients with impairments after a stroke that weren't there before.

79. How can stroke survivors find new activities?

Dr. Monroe: Identify your strengths, as well as your goals. Then find recreational activities you can do independently or with a little support that make use of those strengths. As you engage in these activities successfully, you'll build confidence and motivation to try other new things.

Ask yourself what you enjoy doing. If you have a good recreational therapist, he or she can find a way to get you back into any activity that you enjoy doing, or find something very similar that makes use of your abilities and interests. There are modifications you can make to sporting equipment, assistive devices for helping people with mobility, and other creative and low-tech ways to eliminate barriers. It may be that you have to add duct tape to a pencil to make it easier to grip or use a simple wooden card holder so you can play cards with one hand. Computers can be used for socialization and communication if someone isn't able to get out into the community as much.

"I think hobbies are good for people. Sometimes there are ways to adapt that you may not have realized. For example, if you go online and search for "one-handed fishing" or "one-handed crocheting," you will likely find some tips. I have a one-handed card holder to help me play cards. Return to hobbies you used to love, or find new ones. Find hobbies you can still enjoy. These can become part of your therapy." — David

A Tip from Dr. Mike

"David's stroke reminds me of how precious life is and how lucky we are that he is happy and healthy. Perhaps you have a similar experience as a stroke survivor or family member. Don't waste life by zoning out on the couch all day. No matter your current level of ability, take advantage of this precious day. Connect. Enjoy. Stop existing. Start living."

80. What is recreational therapy and how can it help with stroke recovery?

Dr. Monroe: Therapeutic recreation, or recreational therapy, is a whole field of rehabilitation that uses recreation and other activity-based interventions to address the needs of people with illness and/ or disabling conditions. We look at people from a holistic perspective, addressing their physical, cognitive, emotional, social, and leisure needs.

It's a strength-oriented approach, so it's really about focusing on what people *can* do as opposed to focusing on what they *can't* do. Then it's about using those strengths to engage them in activities that they enjoy and then building on their skills.

Most well-established rehabilitation facilities offer recreational therapy. Recreational therapy is not included in the "three-hour rule," which requires facilities to provide three hours of daily physical, occupational, or speech therapy, but recreational therapy can be part of the whole rehabilitative process. We're the youngest of the therapies, so we're still trying to make headway into places. Stroke survivors should ask for it because it has incredible benefits.

When people lose part of their functioning, they don't feel like they can do anything well anymore. Their definition of themselves has been changed because their abilities have changed. It's important to enable them to try things in a safe environment. When you're playing games, it's not that big of a deal if you lose. When people can have fun, they're more likely to do activities.

We work as part of the rehab team. To help with communication, recreational therapy provides opportunities for socialization to take place through group activities, singing, games, and community outings. We use the strategies provided by the speech-language pathologist to help those with communication problems participate. For physical recovery, we work with the physical therapist to learn what exercises or body positions the stroke survivor is working on, and then find activities the person can do to practice those skills.

Every activity that we use is carefully selected to enable clients to practice the skills they need to practice. We identify their strengths to get them engaged in the activities, but then we build on those strengths to develop skills in the areas where there are some weaknesses.

A game like Monopoly may be used to practice fine motor control—learning to grip, move small pieces, or turn over cards. It can be used to target cognitive functioning: When do I buy? When do I sell? Do I need a hotel? How many spaces do I move? We can work on social skills, like knowing when to take a turn and how to react to wins and losses.

Boccie is a fun game that can be played indoors or outdoors. It's really good for things like range of motion, standing balance, and moving around to get the balls back once you've thrown them. If the affected arm has the ability to grip a ball even slightly, we would use the affected side. We constantly remind our survivors that even if the affected side doesn't feel like it's doing much, they should still lift it up and put it on the table to give it sensory input. If the affected side is weak, we will oftentimes provide hand-over-hand assistance to help them use it, or we'll let them use the hand of choice to be more successful. Typically we start using the nonaffected side to get survivors engaged in the activities, and then encourage them to bring the other side into the game. It can be a bit sneaky.

Because people see recreational therapy as just "fun," they sometimes don't want to do it, especially if they're in the early stages of stroke recovery. They're just focused on wanting to walk, dress, or talk. They don't yet understand that these skills transfer and can be practiced in other ways. We make sure people understand the meaning and purpose of our activities, what the goals are, and why we selected the activities. Our hardest job as recreational therapists can be to help people understand that we are not just playing games, but that through these activities, games, or outdoor pursuits they are actually building skills that will enable them to do other things in their lives more effectively.

100 Activities and Hobbies to Consider

It's important to fill your days with meaningful and enjoyable activities to keep your mind and body active. If you're not spending every day at work or in therapy, consider trying a new activity or taking up a hobby you had never had time to pursue. The next time you think, "I'm bored," browse this list for ideas:

1. Acting
2. Audiobooks or podcasts
3. Auto repair
4. Bible study or book clubs
5. Billiards or pool
6. Bird watching
7. Blogging or keeping a journal
8. Board games
9. Boating and sailing
10. Bowling
11. Cake decorating
12. Calligraphy
13. Camping or traveling in an RV
14. Candle or soap making
15. Canning or preserving food
16. Card games (solitaire, poker, bridge)
17. Ceramics, pottery, or sculpture
18. Chatting online
19. Church, synagogue, or mosque
20. Collage or decoupage
21. Collecting (stamps, coins, shells)
22. Computers or technology
23. Cooking or baking
24. Cross-country skiing or snowshoeing
25. Cutting coupons or bargain hunting
26. Cycling
27. Dancing
28. Dog training or walking

29. Dominoes or mahjongg
30. Drawing
31. Embroidery or cross-stitch
32. Environmental cleanup
33. Family and friends
34. Fantasy sports leagues
35. Fishing or hunting
36. Fitness
37. Flower arranging or bonsai
38. Galleries and museums
39. Gardening
40. Genealogy
41. Hair styling or makeup
42. Home-brewing beer
43. Home decorating or improvement
44. Horseback riding
45. Ice-skating or in-line skating
46. Investing
47. Jewelry making
48. Juggling or twirling
49. Kayaking or canoeing
50. Kite flying or Frisbee
51. Knitting, crocheting, or macramé
52. Lawn work
53. Learning foreign languages
54. Magic tricks
55. Making scrapbooks
56. Martial arts including tai chi

57. Meditation
58. Mentoring in Big Brothers/Sisters or Scouts
59. Metal detecting
60. Models
61. Motorcycles
62. Music appreciation and concerts
63. Musical instruments
64. Origami
65. Painting, watercolors, or coloring
66. Photography
67. Playing sports (golf, tennis, team sports)
68. Political advocacy or fund-raising
69. Print making or letter setting
70. Puppetry
71. Puzzles (jigsaw, crossword, Sudoku)
72. Reading
73. Rock climbing or rappelling
74. Role-play games
75. Scuba diving or snorkeling
76. Sewing or quilting
77. Shopping
78. Singing
79. Skiing or snowboarding
80. Sledding or tubing
81. Social media
82. Stained glass making or glassblowing
83. Stand-up comedy or storytelling
84. Surfing the web

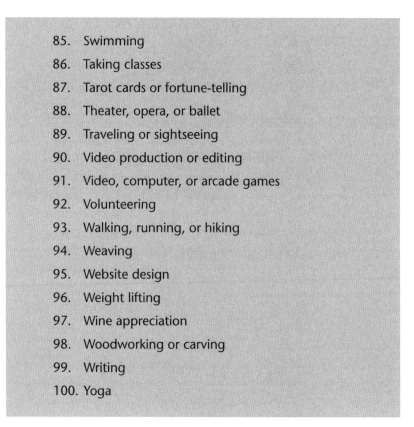

85. Swimming

86. Taking classes

87. Tarot cards or fortune-telling

88. Theater, opera, or ballet

89. Traveling or sightseeing

90. Video production or editing

91. Video, computer, or arcade games

92. Volunteering

93. Walking, running, or hiking

94. Weaving

95. Website design

96. Weight lifting

97. Wine appreciation

98. Woodworking or carving

99. Writing

100. Yoga

81. What is music therapy and how can it help stroke survivors?

Ms. Thompson: Music therapy is the use of music to maximize a person's functioning in different areas of his or her life. Music and music therapy techniques can help stroke survivors improve their communication, sensory/motor functioning, and cognitive abilities. Neuroscientists have long studied how music is processed in the brain, and we've discovered that music is very robust—it tends to stick around in the brain after an injury or stroke, even when other abilities are impaired. Music isn't just one thing; it has rhythm, melody, harmony, and lyrics, among other elements. Each of these is processed differently in the brain. A music therapist uses certain techniques to manipulate those elements of music to create therapeutic change as part of a larger therapy team.

I commonly hear people say, "I'm not good at music. I'm not a musician." I tell people, "Your brain's already hardwired for music. It doesn't matter if you're good at music or not. That's not the goal."

We can use rhythm to help people get more symmetry in their steps for walking. Survivors can learn to adjust the size of their steps to be better able to change speeds and walk in their environment in general. To get the upper extremity moving after a stroke, we can use musical instruments. We might have people reach out to hit a drum, and that drum gives them feedback about how they move. So if they move slowly and hit without a lot of force, they'll hear a light tap on the drum, versus a loud bang, which they would hear if they really punched their arm out there. That is good information to help with *proprioception,* or awareness of where the arm is in space—something that is often damaged by a stroke. We're making use of the auditory system, which works really quickly, to inform the motor system. If people are trying to get fingers moving, then we may use a keyboard or piano to help with that. Essentially we're using instruments to help the brain and arm reconnect and help the brain understand what the outcome of the movement is.

Some people with aphasia can sing entire songs even when they can't otherwise get their words out. It's quite incredible, and it can be very emotional for family members to see their loved ones singing. The music therapist can then work with the speech therapist to help the patients use music as a scaffold for speaking without the music. The music is used to jump-start the brain and form new connections, and often we start to see more spontaneous improvement. With slurred speech, we use rhythm to create more separation between the words so that people can be more clearly understood.

We can also use music to help with attention. A music therapist may have a person listen for certain elements and block out others. Music can help with memory as well, helping people keep steps in order or learn new things. Remember, we all learned the alphabet with a song. Sometimes music therapists will write songs for people around certain procedures or sequences of things that they need to do for daily functioning. For example, a stroke survivor in a wheelchair needs to remember all the steps for transferring to another chair safely. They've got to lock the brakes on their wheelchair, scoot to the edge, stand up, swivel around, and all the other things. Sometimes I get called in by occupational or physical therapists to put together a song with all the steps for someone having difficulty remembering. People remember words in songs a lot better than words without music.

Music therapy can be started as soon as other therapies begin (a few days to a week poststroke). There are benefits to starting early, but music therapy can be helpful at all stages of recovery. You can find music therapists through the American Music Therapy Association (MusicTherapy.org) or through the Certification Board for Music Therapists (cbmt.org). Check local hospitals, outpatient clinics, and stroke support groups to see if there are music therapists providing services. Unfortunately Medicare does not cover music therapy for stroke survivors, but private insurance may pay for music therapy on a case-by-case basis. Health savings accounts or flexible spending accounts can be used to cover music therapy services. In Denver, we work with the local stroke association to offer low-cost group therapy sessions.

Even if you don't have access to music therapy, we can all use music to help us through things when we're not in a good place. A lot of times you find that song with the right words or the right feeling to express what you can't, and it can be so helpful. We can also use music to motivate and lift our spirits. Music with a faster tempo, something upbeat with a good rhythm, can get us moving. If you get the right song, it will perk you up just the same as a cup of coffee. Listen to the music you connect with to match or lift your mood.

• • • • •

Takeaway Points:

A stroke will change your life. You will need to find your new normal. Be patient with yourself. It's okay to make mistakes. You can't do everything perfectly, but could you ever?

Take baby steps to getting back into the community. Go out with support at first; then build your independence as you practice and gain confidence.

Planning is part of the recovery process, and plans may change along the way. Nobody knows what the future holds. Get help in knowing what your options are, and don't put off thinking about finances.

Unfortunately, few stroke survivors return to work. For those who can, work provides therapeutic challenges and gives people purpose. For those who can't, it's important to find another meaningful activity to keep you motivated.

Use your strengths to find recreational activities to keep you engaged. A recreational therapist can help you adapt your hobbies or find new ones.

Music therapy can improve communication, mobility, and cognition through rhythm, melody, and song. You can use the power of music to lift your mood, regulate your walking, or get the words flowing.

CHAPTER 11

RECOVERING YOU

A stroke can and will disrupt your body, thoughts, and activities. But often the most devastating and long-lasting impact it has will be on your spirit. A stroke can strip your confidence. It can fill you with anxiety and sadness. It can make you lose faith in the promise of life, leaving you to question how something like this could ever happen to you. It's this mental battle that's the hardest to win. You'll need to fight hard to stay positive and surround yourself with people who can truly help. This is the part of your recovery where psychologists, social workers, counselors, friends, and even animals can help most.

◇◇

A stroke survivor asks, "Will my life ever be normal again?"

Dr. Woodward: Stroke is a life-changing experience. The trajectory of recovery varies so much from person to person because there are so many complicated factors. The good news is that the majority of stroke survivors reach a point where they can do many of the things that they did before (work, family obligations, social activities, etc.). Things may not be exactly how they were before the stroke, but there certainly is hope for recovery with good therapy and support from family and friends.

Dr. Hinkle: A lot of stroke survivors describe their poststroke life as *a new normal*. Some things may even be better. For example, some people who were fiercely independent learn to accept help from others, and they find that it's a mutually beneficial experience for them. People may feel that they've lost some things, and they have, but they also end up making gains as well. It's going to be different. Nothing ever stays the same—not for anybody.

◇◇

82. How does a stroke change people and relationships?

Dr. Woodward: Stroke can change people and relationships simply because of the stress of the experience. It changes roles. When a wife who runs a household has a stroke, suddenly her husband has to deal with all those household tasks in addition to taking care of his wife. Those role changes can negatively impact people's mental health and their relationships. Damage to the brain can also directly cause physiological changes that lead to personality changes and emotional difficulties.

In some recent focus groups with caregivers and patients, one of the things that caregivers were most surprised about was how their stroke survivor's personality changed. Someone who was very calm and stable beforehand was way more volatile and had more emotional outbursts after the stroke. The caregivers said it was the hardest thing they had to deal with—even harder than having to help the stroke survivor go to the toilet or perform any of those personal-care tasks. It can help to talk about it as part of an ongoing conversation because stroke survivors may not even realize they've changed or what effect the change has on their loved ones. They may benefit from talking with a professional to learn skills to cope with the changes or manage emotions better.

83. How does stroke affect mental health, and how does mental health affect stroke recovery?

Dr. Woodward: Poststroke depression is pretty common, and it comes about for a number of reasons. One is simply that a stroke is a traumatic event. But because stroke affects the brain, it can also be a physiological change that leads to depression. Certainly if people had depression before they had a stroke, or if they have a family history of depression, they're at a much higher risk of experiencing depression after a stroke. Then the circumstances of their recovery can influence poststroke depression as well.

Stroke definitely has an impact on your mental health, and the severity and duration of that impact varies. Poststroke depression can slow recovery in a number of ways. The depression itself makes it really hard for you to engage in the things that you need to do to recover. Anyone who has experienced depression knows how it immobilizes you. Therapy is hard work, but it's so much harder when you're depressed.

The depression can also worsen other things you may experience after a stroke. Pain, as well as fatigue, sleeping problems, and malnutrition, can be worse when you have depression. There are several treatment options, so it's important for survivors, caregivers, and professionals to keep an eye out for depression and talk to a doctor if they notice anything. There can be a stigma attached to mental health problems like depression, so you may be hesitant to speak up. But depression is treatable with medication and counseling, so it's important not to let it get in the way of your best possible recovery.

"I was depressed for a couple of years. I stayed home on the couch, slept a lot, and didn't have friends. It was really hard. When I had something to look forward to, it really improved my mood. I began to travel (cruises are my favorite), and it made me feel like part of the world again. I made friends. I laughed again. It was good for me to try new things. I suggest you engage in activities. Connect with others. Make new friends. Find something you look forward to." — David

A Tip from Dr. Mike

"My brother, my family, and I have found the five stages of grief applied to our own journey. You too may feel you're mourning the prestroke version of yourself or loved one. There are times we were in **denial**, felt **angry**, **bargained**, and felt **depressed**. They're all normal feelings after a stroke. Seek professional help if you need it, or get support from loved ones. By doing so, you may find more **acceptance** in your life."

Guided Visualization: Resilience from Within from Dr. Mike

Resilience is something that can be developed. Guided visualizations can help you become more resilient by tapping into the strength within you. Of course, visualizations can also help you relax when you are feeling stressed. They can provide you with a sense of hope when you are feeling low. They can help you to draw on your inner resources of faith, courage, and strength when you need it most.

They can also help you follow an acronym that wounded soldiers live their lives by: **FOB**. It stands for this:

- **Forward** thinking

- Looking for **opportunities**

- **Building** a new life

Reflect on this for a moment before we begin this visualization.

Now let's do a short guided visualization that can help you enlist your ideal self to take part in your recovery process. Read it to yourself. Or close your eyes as someone reads it to you.

Wherever you are in your life—whether you're in a hospital bed or in your home—just begin by paying attention to where you are now. Feel the air as it's warmed by your nostrils on your next inhalation. And then feel your belly contract as that breath moves out.

Now set an intention for what you'd like to find in this visualization. Are you seeking courage? Strength? Faith? Patience? Speak whatever you're seeking in this moment silently to yourself or, if you'd like, out loud into the universe.

Now, in your mind's eye, see yourself in the most beautiful, peaceful place you've ever been. It can be a place you've actually been to. Your favorite beach. A grassy meadow. Or maybe it's just a heavenly place you're creating for yourself in this moment. Feel the warm air on your cheek. Hear the sound of waves crashing or branches swaying in the breeze. Notice how it feels to take this little mental break as you transport yourself to your own private, happy place.

Blissfully soaking in this precious moment, you soon notice a path in front of you. You have an overwhelming feeling that you are meant to go down this path. You feel peaceful as you begin to walk and can even feel the crunch of the earth with each step you take. Your journey down this path feels light and effortless. You walk with faith that you will reach your destination.

Then you see a clearing up ahead. You feel as though you are meant to move toward this clearing. You soon notice a figure in the distance. As you walk forward, you soon realize that this figure is a person.

As you move closer, you realize this person is you. Only this is no ordinary you. Standing in front you is the most evolved, spiritual, and ideal version of yourself. This ideal you has already attained many of the gains you're working on in your life. He or she is filled with optimism, faith, patience, and resilience. Your ideal self is indeed quite wise, and you realize he or she has a very important piece of advice for you. This advice is quite short—just a few words. And this sentence that you're about to hear holds the key to your receiving a piece of what you are needing today. So with an open heart listen carefully for the wise words your ideal self has for you. Allow this advice to wash over your body, mind, and spirit. Thank your ideal self for those words you needed to hear.

Finally, see you and your ideal self merging together into one physical being. In that moment, realize that your ideal self doesn't live in a faraway place in some imaginary land. The person that is filled with all the patience, faith, and courage you need is already here within you. Whenever you are struggling or at your wit's end, all you need to do is call upon this highest version of yourself to help get you through it. The more you call upon your highest self to guide your actions or support you, the more you become this beautiful, ideal version of yourself. You already have the resilience you need to get through anything life throws at you.

84. How does stress affect brain health and recovery for a stroke survivor?

Dr. Roth: Clearly stress plays a role in recovery, mostly because it takes the focus away from people doing their day-to-day activities. If they're preoccupied with things that are not directly related to what's good and healthy for them and their families, obviously that could be adverse to recovery.

We often use anxiety-reducing activities like yoga, tai chi, imagery, and other psychological interventions. I urge many of our patients to see a psychotherapist. Everyone who goes through a stroke has something to talk about. Talk to someone about it—if not a psychotherapist, then a priest, family member, or somebody. Although I would obviously prefer that you see a professional.

I'm a huge fan of psychotherapy and many of the psychological approaches, though there are many patients for whom medications could be helpful.

◇◇

A stroke survivor says, "I cry really easily now or for no reason. This isn't like me. Why?"

Dr. Chiu: There's a high prevalence of mood disturbance after stroke. It can happen just as readily after a mild stroke, where you have excellent recovery, as it can after a major stroke. So it isn't necessarily what you might think—that people who have had bad strokes and are disabled are always depressed. It isn't as simple as that, because there are changes in brain chemistry that occur after a stroke, and there's a very strong link between this alteration of neurochemistry and disturbances of mood. About a third of patients will experience depression or anxiety at some point after a stroke.

However, there's also a condition called *pseudobulbar affect,* also known as *emotional lability,* which is not exactly depression. People with pseudobulbar affect will cry suddenly, or sometimes they will laugh suddenly, for apparently no reason. If you ask those people why they started crying, they might say, "I don't know. I wasn't feeling sad." In depression, the person will tell you they feel sad or blue, but in a patient with pseudobulbar affect, there is a disassociation between the internal mood and what comes out. It used to be called *emotional incontinence,* and it's sometimes seen in patients who've had a stroke.

All of these mood disorders—depression, pseudobulbar affect, anxiety—are treatable. So if you recognize them, be upfront with your doctor and let him or her know. We know that mood disorders, particularly depression, can hold back someone's recovery from a stroke and we don't want that to happen.

◇◇

85. How do communication problems affect one's mental health?

Dr. Hinckley: Self-esteem and self-image are often affected. A person who suddenly has aphasia after a stroke has to reconstruct who they are and how they are dealing with the world and functioning in it. It's not a short or easy process.

When you have a sudden loss of any ability—particularly a communication ability—you are going to go through a **grieving process**. It's important to acknowledge that while you have survived, you have also lost a lot. It's okay to grieve for those losses.

Just like in any grieving process, there is a risk of depression that might persist over time. In fact, the stroke itself can put somebody at risk for depression because of changes in the brain. Depression is a very serious issue for those who've had a stroke. If it's left untreated, the person might be less likely to engage in therapy or any kind of positive or productive activity, which therefore stops improvement. Often this ends up in a vicious cycle because the person sees they're not improving and it leads them to a deeper depression. It's very important to pay attention to mental health issues after stroke, not just for the person with aphasia, but also for the family members or caregivers who are living with that person.

People with aphasia are at a higher risk of depression than other stroke survivors. However, going to talk with a counselor is one of the greatest difficulties for people with aphasia for two reasons. One is their own difficulty in being able to express what their concerns and experiences are. Second, there aren't many mental health professionals who are trained to support or accommodate that communication difficulty. In my practice, I have had great difficulty finding a counselor or mental health professional who is willing to work with a person with aphasia in individual counseling, because those professionals are not aware of what communication strategies or techniques to use to help bridge the communcation gap so they can engage in the counseling. I have gone in as the speech-language pathologist to meet with a counselor and a person with aphasia during the first session solely to demonstrate and to make sure they are comfortable with the communication strategies that the two of them can use. Usually after one session the counselor can continue with using those strategies. It's possible to train people with general strategies, but this individualized approach is probably the most effective.

Finding Therapy That Works for You from Dr. Mike

Many stroke survivors experience depression. Traditional talk therapy like cognitive behavioral therapy (CBT) may be difficult for survivors dealing with communication issues. Innovative therapy models may help ease depression for people with aphasia or any stroke survivor who struggles with counseling or talk therapy. Look for guided CBT self-help workbooks you can complete at your own pace (with help if needed). Therapists with education in art or music therapy are trained to facilitate communication and process emotions in nonverbal ways.

Mindfulness meditation, mindfulness-based stress reduction (MBSR), and mindfulness-based cognitive therapy (MBCT) use guided meditations that don't require much talking. Dr. Jon Kabat-Zinn's MBSR is used in university hospitals around the world, and you can download his meditations onto your phone or computer at MindfulnessApps.com. There are many other good meditation apps available as well, like Headspace and Buddhify. Another form of therapy that combines CBT and mindfulness is called *acceptance and commitment therapy* (ACT). The guided ACT self-help workbook called *Get Out of Your Mind and Into Your Life* is a helpful tool you can read and complete on your own or with guidance.

86. How can stroke survivors stay hopeful?

Dr. Woodward: Having **plans and goals for the future** gives you something to work toward and look forward to. Having friends and family who are also invested in your recovery can also be a strong motivator since you want to do well for the other people in your life.

Listening to other people's stories can help you realize **you're not alone**. Reading stories on stroke websites or hearing from others in peer support groups can give you a sense of "I can do that too," or "This stroke doesn't have to be the end of my life." Other people have come through this and done amazing things.

There are times when you have to focus on the end goal to stay hopeful, but sometimes the task of stroke recovery seems too big and daunting. These are the times when you're better off focusing on the details. Find something that's going right, like "I walked five extra steps today—that's better than I did yesterday." It's important to keep things in perspective and find a good balance between being in the moment and thinking about the future.

> *"When I was little, I wanted to be a doctor. I really felt I had to have a college degree and tried taking some college classes. It was really challenging. I learned a lot, and it was a good experience. My aphasia made it impossible to complete, but I'm glad I tried. Success means trying. Failing is failing to try. You may have a different experience or a different goal, but it's important that you keep trying. If you're trying, you're succeeding."* — David

A Tip from Dr. Mike

"I get really excited about the way we all have the power to improve our brains. Challenging experiences, learning new information, meditation, and exercise all have the power to make the brains actually bigger—just like dumbbell curls pump up biceps. Eating seafood, olive oil, and berries can protect the brain and prevent disease. What's something challenging or healthy you can do today to take care of your most precious organ?"

87. Is there a point where a stroke survivor should give up on therapy and accept that this is how life is going to be?

Dr. Woodward: There certainly can be diminishing returns with therapy. The greatest recovery usually happens in a relatively short period of time, but people still make gains years down the road. **Giving up guarantees that you're not going to improve.** Maybe you can stop focusing on therapy for a while, and if something changes, you can go back and work on it some more. If you make some progress and it stalls out, then maybe you can focus on something else for a while.

Recovery is influenced by so many factors in our lives—it's a moving target. Circumstances can change, and our bodies change over time. It's probably worth always looking at ways to improve, but without therapy becoming an obsession that keeps you from doing other things in your life. **It's a delicate balance of being hopeful, having realistic expectations, and living your life.** Conversations with health professionals can help you understand what those realistic expectations are before you make the decision to say, "Okay, I'm done."

88. It seems that some people identify as *stroke survivors*, others call themselves *stroke victims*, while others use the term *stroke warriors*. Some people celebrate the anniversary of their stroke, whereas others never want to think about it. How important is the language people use and their attitude about their stroke?

Dr. Woodward: Language is how we define ourselves and how we define our experiences. I have a more negative reaction to *stroke victim* than to *stroke survivor,* but some people have the opposite reaction, thinking that if you're a victim, it implies that you didn't do anything wrong—it wasn't your fault. So while the language is important, our interpretations and understanding of that language is important too. We have to honor the way individuals want to talk about themselves. Some people are going to feel really sad on the anniversary of their stroke, and others want to celebrate their recovery. Whichever is the case, we should give them whatever support and attention they need in that moment.

89. Where can people find support for living with stroke?

Dr. Monroe: I recommend support groups, both for the stroke survivor and for the family members. Part of going through something like a stroke is experiencing a sense of isolation and loneliness, thinking that nobody else has to deal with this. **Support groups not only provide socialization, but also help you learn new tricks.** "You can't roll a rolling pin? Well this is what I did to modify my rolling pin, so now I can use it." "You're having trouble getting to the library? This is the person you should contact." Support groups are wonderful places for gaining from the experience of others and not having to learn everything yourself.

Dr. Woodward: I'm a big advocate of peer support because knowing people who have been through similar experiences is key to being able to cope with all of the different things you have to manage on a day-to-day basis. Support groups are great places to get information and find emotional support by talking to people who understand what you're going through. There are a number of face-to-face support groups, as well as many online groups. Often hospitals will manage groups through their stroke centers, and the National Stroke Association website has a database you can search for groups in your area.

◇◇

A stroke survivor asks, "I'm not recovering like the others in my support group. Am I doing something wrong? Should I be comparing myself to others?"

Dr. Woodward: It's human nature to compare ourselves to others. It's hard not to. The benefit of comparing yourself to others is that you get to learn from their experiences and talk to people who have gone through a similar experience. As much as your friends and family try to relate, they haven't gone through a stroke and don't fully understand. Support from people who have experienced a stroke is really important, as long as you keep in mind that you can learn from each other's experiences but that it's not going to be exactly the same.

Every stroke is different, and every stroke survivor is different, and therefore every recovery will be vastly different. People have strokes at different ages, and they may have other health conditions and different resources in terms of accessing care services. There are so many variables that impact how quickly you recover. You can't know all those factors, nor can you control them, so it won't help you to compare.

◇◇◇

A Tip from Dr. Mike

"Human beings sometimes make upward comparisons, comparing themselves to people who seemingly have it better than they do right now—such as people who haven't just had a stroke. This can make us feel discouraged. Instead of comparing yourself to others, focus only on all the positive changes you see in *your* recovery. The most important race isn't with someone else—it's with yourself."

90. Many stroke survivors find that their friends start to disappear. How can stroke survivors retain their friendships or find new social circles?

Dr. Monroe: Stroke survivors may not be comfortable with themselves at first—with how they look or what they can do. When friends want to be involved, the survivors may isolate themselves, telling friends to wait until they're better, or back to normal. Then, because friends think that the person doesn't want to be around them, they pull back.

Another possibility is that friends don't know what to do. They see their friend who has had a stroke, and it makes them feel more vulnerable. They may not know how to interact with people with disabilities. Unfortunately, our society doesn't train people in this area very well. People think, "I can't use a sense of humor because this person has had a stroke." So they change their whole conversation style around you and get all serious. That's not fun. We still need humor and still need to be loved.

So first it's a matter of getting comfortable with yourself and what your skills are, and then if your friends have moved away because of discomfort or other reasons, you need to start reaching out to them. Reach out to connect in places that will be comfortable for everyone. Invite them to your home, or go to a movie to ease back into the relationship. The most important thing is to give people permission to ask questions about your abilities and your needs, and then to let them know how you could use their assistance and where you don't need it.

◇◇◇

A stroke survivor asks, "What happened to my friends? They all sent cards and came to visit me in the hospital, but they are all gone now when I actually need the help and support."

Dr. Woodward: That's not uncommon after any sort of traumatic event. Family and friends, but particularly friends, are there in the moment of the crisis, and then over time they drift back into their normal lives while you're still dealing with the aftermath of everything that has happened. It's not that they don't care or that they aren't thinking about you; most of the time they just don't really know how to help. In a crisis we know to visit people, send cards, and bring flowers. Immediately after you return home, your friends might bring food or call. But in the longer process of recovery, people just aren't quite sure what to do.

It's important to ask for help. If you can't ask for help yourself, find one or two trusted friends who can help organize that support for you. They can contact people and say, "Hey, he's home from the hospital now and needs somebody to come by and spend the afternoon with him because he can't get out of the house," or "She needs transportation to a whole bunch of doctors' appointments over the next couple of weeks, so can we add you to the schedule to help?" Not everybody will stick around, but a good core group of people will usually step up and actually be relieved that you asked. Many of them probably want to help, but don't know what to do and are afraid of intruding or getting in your way during a difficult time.

◇◇◇◇◇◇◇◇◇◇◇◇◇◇◇◇◇◇◇◇◇◇◇◇◇◇◇◇◇◇◇◇◇◇◇◇◇◇◇

91. Can pets help stroke survivors?

Dr. Monroe: Absolutely! Pets are great for stroke survivors or anybody with a disability. Pets provide companionship, socialization, and unconditional love. Some pets can even be trained to assist stroke survivors in doing things they're no longer able to do. It also gives the survivors an opportunity to do something meaningful and have purpose in their lives through taking care of the pet by feeding and grooming it. If you have a dog, it will need to be walked, and that can be a good way to practice your walking skills, as long as the dog's not too strong for you. The companionship of a pet can certainly help to decrease the loneliness that is often felt when people have a stroke.

> "When I was growing up, we had a dog. It was such a relief to come home after school and have my dog waiting for me. He'd get so excited to see me and didn't care that I couldn't speak well. It really helped with my mood and self-esteem. I could also try talking to him without being afraid of making a mistake. Today, my dog Sebastian always puts a smile on my face. If you don't have one, a pet or service animal can be something to consider." — David

> ## A Tip from Dr. Mike
>
> "Sometimes stroke survivors are abandoned by their old friends. But you may be surprised by how faithful other friends are throughout this process. One thing is certain: friendship and companionship are essential for all human beings. Try your best to strengthen the friendships you have while simultaneously cultivating new ones. Companionship is the antidote to isolation and loneliness."

92. What is mindfulness and how can it help stroke survivors?

Dr. Monroe: Mindfulness is being in the present moment, fully and completely, and not reflecting on the past, which leads to a lot of regrets or worrying about the future. It's about bringing your awareness to what's happening, and not letting your thoughts take control.

I created a program called the BREATH Pathway, which we use at the Center for Life Skills. It's a conceptual model that can help you recognize and eliminate stressors and negative influences in your life, while helping you to experience joy.

Breathing: Focusing on how it can affect you physiologically as well as emotionally.

Responsibility: It's ultimately our choice about how we're going to respond to certain situations. Do you get angry when people are rude, or do you educate them?

Environment: Being aware of which environments make you uncomfortable, feel more at peace with yourself, and enable you to practice your skills better.

Awareness: Knowing what's happening in and around you now.

Thankfulness: Sometimes we forget that even if bad things have happened to us, there's a lot of good in our lives.

Habits: Be aware of the way you habitually do things, and find new ways of reacting to situations you are faced with.

A Mindfulness Meditation for Survivors and Loved Ones from Dr. Mike

Mindfulness and mindfulness meditation can be valuable tools for stroke survivors and their loved ones. By definition, mindfulness is simply paying attention to the present moment without judgment or reaction. It's just noticing what is happening in the moment.

It can help us avoid getting caught up in anxieties about the future so that we feel more peaceful in day-to-day life—especially in the moments that are difficult or anxiety inducing. Mindfulness can improve our moods and is even used to treat depression. Right here and right now are the only things you need to worry about—no matter where you are in your recovery journey. So make a decision to **be here now**.

Mindfulness is helpful for stroke survivors and their loved ones in specific ways:

- For stroke survivors, mindfulness can help you to tolerate the anxiety you feel when you are communicating or completing a task. Instead of judging yourself, becoming embarrassed, and letting others do the talking for you, you can get the time and space to find and speak the word you're looking for through mindful awareness. Take a breath. Slow down. Focus on what you're doing—one syllable or movement at a time—without judgment.

- For loved ones, mindfulness can teach you to tolerate the feelings of anxiety you may feel when a stroke survivor is searching for a word or taking a little extra time to complete a task. You instinctively may want to finish a survivor's sentence or do everything for your loved one. And while this comes from a good place with kind intent, *overhelping* can actually hurt survivors in the long run since it prevents them from having the opportunity do something that increases neuroplasticity. Sometimes, we need to give stroke survivors time to complete a sentence or task themselves. This can lead to long-term gains in speech and movement. Don't let your own anxiety hinder their recovery journey.

Here's a brief **mindfulness meditation on sounds** that you can do wherever you are. You can either read it as your practice or have someone read it to you.

Wherever you are right now, take a moment to settle into your body and just notice where you are. Feel your feet. Sense your breath. See the color on the backs of your eyelids. Just notice. Just watch. Simply become aware of what's going on right here and right now.

If you notice thoughts, feelings, or sensations throughout this practice, just notice them without judgment. You can just acknowledge them with a quick "Oh, there's anxiety again," or "Hello, planning," or "I see you, worry." Just let them all be there—just as they are—without pushing them away.

Now, turn your attention to your sense of sound. First, find the nearest sound you can detect—such as the beating of your heart or the sound of your breath. Next, find the farthest and faintest sound you can detect in this moment. Imagine that you're not just hearing with your ears; you're hearing with your entire body. The sounds that are near you and sounds that are far away. Loud sounds and soft sounds. In this practice, just notice sounds without judging or labeling them—even if they're sounds you'd usually judge as pleasant or unpleasant. Perceive all sounds simply as pure waves of energy and sensation.

Now pay special attention not just to sounds but also to the spaces between sounds. Let the spaces linger as you notice any reactions in your body. Just allow the sounds and spaces between them to linger without doing anything at all. Just listen. Just be. Notice how good it feels not to have to do anything in the silence.

Now, notice this nonreactive and focused attention you've cultivated in this moment. In your mind's eye, picture yourself as the speaker having a conversation. See and hear yourself mindfully taking your time with each sound and word. There's no rush. There's only this moment. This is especially helpful for stroke survivors, but it's a lesson we all need to remember.

Next, see yourself having a conversation with someone. See and hear yourself receiving their syllables and words—and the spaces between them—without having to do anything. Notice any anxious energy you may have—just notice that energy. Use this mindful awareness to become a container that holds that energy. This is especially helpful for loved ones, but it's also helpful for stroke survivors when they talk to other survivors.

Take this kind of awareness you've cultivated during this meditation, and imagine yourself infusing your daily life with this moment-by-moment, breath-by-breath, step-by-step, and sound-by-sound mindfulness. You can add this present-moment awareness to everything that you do in your daily life in the only moment where your life is unfolding. Just here. Just now.

• • • • •

Takeaway Points:

Change is inevitable. Hope and optimism can help you handle it. Be prepared for big changes in your relationships, and perhaps even in your personality.

Poststroke depression, anxiety, and stress are extremely common, but help is available. Your recovery will go more smoothly if you manage these mental health conditions rather than ignore them. People with aphasia are at a higher risk for depression than other stroke survivors, and they have fewer ways to talk about their feelings. If your loved one has aphasia, be particularly aware of his or her mood and seek help if needed.

Hope is powerful. Stay hopeful by having plans and goals for the future. Build a strong support network of people who truly care and understand what you're going through.

Attend stroke support groups in your community to learn from others, but do not compare yourself. Remember, every stroke is different and every stroke survivor is unique. Just do your best in your own life and circumstances.

Friends come and go throughout our lives, but they especially seem to go after a stroke. Not everyone is strong enough to see you struggle. Ask your friends for help with specific tasks so they will feel useful, and find things you all enjoy doing.

Consider adding a furry friend to your life for extra companionship. Caring for a pet can give you purpose and get you moving.

Mindfulness is a process of focusing your attention on the present moment rather than focusing on regrets or worries. Stroke survivors can benefit from learning to be in the moment and connecting with their breath. Appreciate what you do have, and find joy where you can.

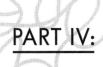

PART IV:

YOUR FAMILY
&
YOUR FUTURE

CHAPTER 12

CAREGIVER CONCERNS

A stroke doesn't affect just one person; it affects the person's family and friends as well. There's often one person in the stroke survivor's life (a spouse, parent, grown child, sibling, or friend) who steps up and takes responsibility to become the primary caregiver. This is usually a new role for this person, and it comes with new challenges. Family caregiving is often unpaid and underappreciated, but it is an essential service that we provide to the people we love when they are in need. Stroke recovery can take a very long time, so caregivers have to be prepared for the hard work and long road ahead.

93. How can caregivers best help with recovery?

After putting this question to many of our experts, we heard three prevailing themes:

1. Be supportive, but encourage independence.
2. Take care of yourself too.
3. Don't do it alone. Accept help.

Let's start with the first one: be supportive, but encourage independence.

Dr. Ploughman: Early on, when a person has just had a stroke, family members can help by sitting and interacting with that person on the affected side. Encourage the person to look to the affected side, and touch the person on the affected side. This helps with awareness, plasticity, and activity on that affected side.

Later, family members or caregivers can help with the exercises, learning what the therapists want the stroke survivor to do. You will often find that therapists have many jobs for family members to do, like practicing range-of-motion exercises or assisting the person with the stroke in practicing balance and walking. It's very important to do those extra repetitions to maximize early recovery.

Dr. Page: Families can help with exercises and make sure the stroke survivors stay vigilant with their therapies. Home exercises are so important for a lot of different reasons. They help not only with restoration of function but also with maintaining range of motion and any function the patient still has. Family members are also important for things such as transporting patients to appointments and making sure that stroke survivors get out into the community.

Challenging loved ones is also important for family members. Sometimes family members don't challenge their loved ones enough. It's hard for a son to challenge his dad, to tell him to do his exercises or to speak more slowly. But a lot of times that's exactly what patients need—some really tough love to push through. Stroke recovery is not for wimps. It's dedicated practice, and it takes millions of attempts to change the brain and cause the arm or the leg or the speech to recover. That happens, in part, through the help of a motivated caregiver.

Dr. Hinckley: Whenever possible we have to let our loved ones do things for themselves. When people have strokes, they become patients. In the hospital, the nurse comes in and does things for them. Everybody does things for them because they are sick or can't talk well. There has to be a transition from receiving total care to getting back to an independent life. So once your loved one is at home, you have to **ask the person what he wants help with, instead of just doing it for him**. He has to start taking ownership of himself and his situation.

Dr. Monroe: Be patient and supportive, but don't do too much. It's hard to see loved ones struggle. It can be very difficult to see loved ones not performing, looking, or acting the way we are used to seeing them. However, it's important not to do too much for them, because it doesn't help in the long run. They have to struggle to learn the new skills. **It's not only about skill development; it's also about confidence**—the knowledge that they can do things themselves and don't have to depend on other people. It's important to allow people to speak for themselves and to give them the time to do it and the time to find the mechanisms through which they can do it.

Now, let's see what the experts had to say about the second theme: Take care of yourself too.

Dr. Hinckley: The burden of caregiving is very great, and it increases health risks and problems. Finding a balance in this new life of living with a stroke survivor is critical. **Don't let yourself get in the position of being burned out and at the end of your rope.** It's important to find good ways of coping.

Dr. Woodward: Caregivers tend to neglect themselves and often feel guilty for taking time for themselves or looking out for themselves. You know the little safety spiel they give on airplanes about securing your oxygen mask before helping someone else? I think that is very analogous to this circumstance. **You can't be a good caregiver if you're not taking care of yourself.** You have to recognize when you need help. You can't be afraid to ask for help.

The Administration on Aging offers the National Family Caregiver Support Program, which provides a number of support options for caregivers, including *respite care*. This is temporary professional care that gives caregivers a break. Many people don't realize respite care is available, or they delay getting it until they are so burned out that they don't get the full benefit from it. It's better to get respite care early on, before you feel like you really need it, in order to be able to maintain your health. The program can refer you for counseling and help you figure out how to get supplemental services. Sometimes they can help with home improvements, medical supplies, or legal assistance, so it's a good resource to look into. (More information can be found in Appendix A at the end of this book.)

And the final theme: Don't do it alone. Accept help.

Dr. Hinkle: One of the most important things for stroke survivors and caregivers to do is to accept the help people offer. If people ask, "What can we do?" think of something specific for them to do. Can they go grocery shopping for you? Can they drive the stroke survivor to an appointment? Walk the dog? **Let them do things if they offer.**

Dr. Hinckley: Make a list of specific things that would help you and that you can ask family members or friends or neighbors to help you with, and don't be afraid to ask for assistance. Ask others to take the stroke survivor out shopping or to an event. You don't have to carry the whole burden yourself. In fact, if you do, it's likely to be detrimental.

It's often very difficult for caregivers to help with home programs and practice. None of us wants his or her significant other to be a therapist; we want that person to be in the role of spouse or partner. It's hard to take on extra roles, and often it doesn't work well. The solution is to **recruit somebody who can come over on a set schedule to do that home practice with the stroke survivor**. It could be a neighbor, friend, or volunteer from your place of worship. Put home exercises on the list of things you can ask somebody else to help you with. Friends or neighbors may actually be thrilled to have something concrete like that to help with. In my experience, most stroke survivors respond better when practicing with somebody else than when practicing with the immediate caregiver. Don't feel guilty about it; just get someone else to help you.

"My mom and I lived in the hospital for three months. She slept in a chair next to my bed. Most of the time, she didn't look good. I remember feeling better when she finally started to put makeup on, because I knew it meant she was starting to take care of

herself again. When we got home, my mom created a team to help me. Being a caregiver was a full-time job for her. A neighbor came over to do exercises with me. Sometimes we played a game. People from church brought food. My friend Kelly came over a lot, and we always laughed together. She was the one friend who stuck by me, and she is still my good friend 20 years later. My mom brought in a watercolor teacher for me. Painting was therapeutic, and it was something I learned to do really well with one hand. When people offered help, my mom took it."
— David

A Tip from Dr. Mike

"Here's a common dynamic I see in families I have treated: Caretakers feel burned out but feel guilty if they take a break when there's just so much work to do. Stroke survivors sense this and also feel guilty; this makes them feel like their needs are too overwhelming. This is a lose-lose situation for both caretakers and survivors. The win-win that worked for my family and the families I have worked with was this: love and take care of yourself. By doing so, you can love and take care of others more."

94. What questions should stroke survivors and families ask before coming home from the hospital?

Dr. Hinkle: You should know your diagnosis, whether you had an ischemic stroke or a hemorrhagic stroke, and what was done to treat the stroke. You should know whether you got the clot-busting drug tPA right after your stroke, since some stroke centers won't allow you to get it again but some will. You should also ask what your risk factors were: "Why did I have this stroke?" The number-one risk factor for stroke is high blood pressure, so if you do have high blood pressure, know your numbers. If the team thinks that the blood pressure was the most likely cause of the stroke, you'll likely be coming home on a new medication.

Know the signs and symptoms of another stroke. Remember the acronym FAST—Face, Arms, and Speech. Test all three, and then it's Time to call for help. Most hospitals will give you the information verbally, but make sure they also give you written information so you have something to refer back to. You're not always absorbing all the information, because it's such a stressful time. Ask a lot of questions and educate yourself as much as possible.

Dr. Woodward: When you're getting ready to leave the hospital, you should be given a discharge plan, so ask lots of questions about that and write down whom to call. A lot of the information the hospital tells you goes in one ear and out the other because it's a chaotic time and people are scared and stressed.

You need to make sure that you understand the details of your discharge plan, including where you're being sent, how long you're going to be there if you're not going home, and what follow-up appointments you need to make. Make sure you know whom to call if you're home and don't remember the answers to those questions or if new questions come up.

◇◇◇

A caregiver says, "I'm struggling in my relationship. Sometimes I'm not sure I can be a caregiver *and* a loved one. Is this normal?"

Dr. Woodward: The long answer is that the experience of stroke is hard on relationships. It's really stressful and brings about a wide range of experiences, emotions, and expectations. Even a relationship that was rock solid before can have some rocky moments after a stroke.

Recovery is a long process, and stroke survivors change—not just from the trauma of the experience, but also possibly physiologically. There can be damage to the brain that causes personality changes, making the survivor seem like a different person. The caregiver also experiences stress, and roles in the relationship change. The whole experience may alter what each person wants out of life. It's an intense experience that has a profound impact on people.

Author's note: Relationships evolve and change, and this is certainly true after a stroke. It's normal for the initial period of adjustment to be difficult and confusing. Sometimes stroke survivors don't make a full recovery, and in these cases, it's vital to find ways to stay connected. Couples who have been together for years sometimes don't need words to understand what each other is thinking or feeling and can find connection in nonverbal ways. The time you've shared together becomes the foundation for a new chapter in your relationship.

Roles may change, and even personalities may change. Talk about what's going on. Seek professional counseling—as a couple or individually—to help you make sense of this new experience. There are some people who leave relationships after a stroke, and this is a fact of life. Exiting a relationship is not unique to people in stroke situations, and the reasons for a relationship ending are often complex. However, there are also people who find a new sense of richness in the poststroke relationship.

◇◇

95. When is it a good idea to consider moving a stroke survivor to a care facility?

Dr. Roth: The decision of where a person will live after a stroke is very individual and based on so many factors. It's important for the family and the patient to be realistic about things and make sure they get the proper supervision and care. If, for example, the person is at risk for falling and sufficient supervision cannot be provided in the home, then the person is at a much greater risk living at home than in a facility.

The idea is to weigh the important factors: risk of complications, medical stability, and the need for day-to-day care, such as bladder and bowel care, dressing, getting out of bed, and mobility. If a family member either can't be around or lacks the ability to manage the care needs, the best decision is to have the stroke survivor live in an environment where there is sufficient care provided. I've seen many families struggle with this, and I totally understand why they would, but it's important to be not only **realistic, but also thoughtful about the patient**. That means making sure the person has enough care.

Dr. Hinkle: For a stroke survivor to go to a nursing home is not a failure. About 25 percent of older people who have had a stroke go to a nursing home. If the caregiver can't do everything and doesn't have the resources, the stroke survivor is going to get better care in a place where there are professionals whose job is to provide care for them.

There are all levels of nursing homes or care facilities. Some people go to a *skilled nursing facility* (SNF), where the staff provides daily therapy until the stroke survivor is able to go home. If a person has had a hemorrhagic stroke, the time line for getting better can be particularly longer, as these survivors tend to make slower gains in their rehabilitation. SNFs can be the best places to allow that healing to happen over time.

Caregiver Tips from Carol Dow-Richards

I'm Carol Dow-Richards, and I'm the proud mother of Mike and David Dow. I know firsthand what it feels like to be a family member and caretaker of a stroke survivor. As a founding board member of the Aphasia Recovery Connection, I frequently speak to caregivers and stroke survivors, offering hope and practical advice.

As a caregiver, you probably feel a lot of loss. Financial security may change. I had to give up my business. Overnight, we went from having two incomes in our household to having just one. Roles may change. Personalities may change.

As your whole life is turned upside down, it is normal and healthy to grieve for what was. I struggled for many years. Looking back on my experiences, I suggest these tips for new stroke caregivers:

1. Take care of yourself too. Many of us make the mistake of wearing ourselves down, and then we're of no help to anyone. So try to get enough sleep, take time for yourself, and see a doctor if anxiety or depression sets in. It is not easy. The worry, fear, and grief can be overwhelming for the caregivers as well as the stroke survivors. Seek help earlier rather than later.

2. When someone calls and says, "Let me know what I can do," give them a job. Don't take this on alone. Family and friends often want to help, but they need your direction. It might be as simple as asking them to run to the store for you, or to sit with your loved one while you run an errand.

3. Learn as much as you can from doctors, therapists, books, and reputable Internet resources. However, don't believe everything you read online. I've known survivors who have paid thousands of dollars for experimental treatments they could barely afford and that ended up being a huge waste of time and money. Your doctors are well versed in treatments that are backed up by research. Ask questions. Ask for advice. Attend the therapy sessions and appointments so you can learn too. I often suggest to caregivers that they use their phones to record some of the exercises that experts suggest to use in at-home practice. It is so easy to forget when the stress level is high.

4. Remember: No two people or strokes are ever exactly alike, so don't compare to others. Learn from others instead. You can meet other families online or through a local support group. It is helpful to

share your experiences and challenges. Knowing you aren't the only one can be helpful.

5. Keep hope alive—even if someone tries to steal it away. Hold hope tight, both for yourself and your stroke survivor. I always believed in David and in the ability of the brain to heal—even when some doctors left me feeling hopeless. I had to keep hope alive. Without hope there's no reason for us to give it our all in the recovery process.

6. Guard your loved one's energy while in the hospital. Limit the number of visitors and the length of time they stay if fatigue is an issue. Try to make sure your loved one is at his or her best and on time for rehab appointments. Rehab appointments are such a valuable commodity in recovery. Do your best to have your loved one rested before the appointment so they can participate and get the most out of the session. Being exhausted during therapy limits the effectiveness and can waste some of that valuable time.

7. Validate your loved one's feelings. Don't discount his or her fear, sadness, or loss. While we tried to be positive around David, it was also important to face the feelings we all had. It's okay to cry and to grieve. Talking about feelings and working through them worked best for our family.

8. Find ways to limit frustration. Find ways to help your stroke survivor adapt to the limitations so he or she can be more independent. Because David could not speak, it was helpful to have a clipboard with paper or some drawing tools nearby. Apps on smartphones and tablets can help with this as well.

9. Stay organized. Use a binder or smartphone to keep track of medical history, prescriptions, insurance information, recommendations, and phone numbers. Check to see when your health insurance's limits reset. You may have run out of therapy coverage

for this calendar year or quarter, but you may get 20 more sessions next year or month. When you're allotted more sessions, use them. Check your out-of-pocket maximums and deductibles. If you've reached your out-of-pocket maximum for the year, it may be beneficial to see specialists or receive any treatments you need this year rather than wait until the next one. If a treatment is not initially preapproved by your insurance, you can sometimes file an appeal. A doctor or therapist can write a letter that can help you make your case with insurance companies and help turn an initial denial into an approval if medical necessity is proven.

10. Remember that you have a relationship beyond the caregiver-patient relationship. Make time for the activities you enjoyed before the stroke to keep those roles alive.

• • • • •

Takeaway Points:

Caregivers can help best with recovery by doing these three things:

1. Be supportive, but encourage independence.

2. Take care of yourself too.

3. Don't do it alone. Give people specific tasks when they offer to help.

Before you leave the hospital, it's important to know:

1. Why your loved one had the stroke

2. What was done to treat it

3. What the discharge plan is

4. Whom to call with questions

If you're having trouble adjusting to your new role as a caregiver, talk about it with your survivor and seek professional help if needed. It's normal to struggle. The person who had the stroke isn't the only one whose life has changed.

While everyone wants to come home after a stroke, there are times to consider care facilities as a temporary or permanent discharge location. Consider whether the care needs are too great to manage at home or if better care is available at a residential care facility. You can always reevaluate your decision.

CHAPTER 13

THE NEXT CHAPTER IN STROKE RECOVERY

While we have learned a great deal about stroke and the brain in the past several decades, there is still so much we don't know. Researchers around the world are making huge discoveries and exploring exciting new treatments for brain repair. Some of these advances are already in use in research clinics, while others are still undergoing safety or funding approval for widespread use. More are still in development but hold huge promise for helping stroke survivors 5 to 10 years down the road. Our experts are on the cutting edge of stroke recovery and share with us their vision of the future. Dr. Dylan Edwards of Burke Rehabilitation Hospital, a physical therapist and leading researcher in robotics, joins our other experts to share his knowledge about the promise of future stroke treatments.

96. What is the future of stroke recovery?

Dr. Chiu: There have been huge advances in the last couple of decades in both stroke prevention and acute-stroke treatment. These have been so successful that we've seen a dramatic drop in stroke mortality rates. In the first few hours after a stroke, we have a window of opportunity to use interventions like tPA (the clot-busting drug) and mechanical clot retrieval. These are things that can make a difference, but they have to be implemented almost immediately.

The big gap in the field right now is in the area of stroke recovery. A lot of people will say, "My doctor always talks to me about things I can do to prevent a stroke, but what do I do about the stroke that I had a month ago, a year ago, five years ago?" And quite honestly, for many years it looked pretty grim. I'm now seeing tremendous promise with the types of stroke recovery therapies we might be talking about in the future—in just a few years. I've been a stroke neurology specialist for 20 years, and this is the first time that I really feel tremendous optimism that we might be on the doorstep of something big in stroke recovery.

Dr. Roth: At the end of the day, what's most important is to recognize that it's likely going to be a cocktail of all these great advances. **It's going to be a combination of brain stimulation with cell therapy, along with exercise and robotic devices.** We don't yet know how much of each or the timing, but that's going to be what's most important in the rehabilitation process in the future of stroke recovery.

97. What is robotic therapy?

Dr. Roth: When we think about technology, we make a distinction between *assistive technology* and *therapeutic technology*. **Assistive technology allows the individual to interface better with his or her environment.** For example, a wheelchair is assistive technology because it allows the person to be mobile in the community. Certain electronic devices that open curtains or answer the phone when you speak or push a button are assistive technology. These are compensations.

Therapeutic technology is where a person operates robotic arms or legs, so **the robotic device is actually helping to strengthen the primary function.** It's actually making the person stronger or helping the person walk with better balance. These are important approaches, and while they're not fully implemented in rehab yet, we're seeing them used more.

Dr. Edwards: Robot-assisted therapy is not science fiction. You can think of robot-assisted therapy as a piece of equipment you might find in a gym or health club. It's a powered device that attaches to a patient, has advanced controllers, and interacts in real time with the capabilities of the person it's exercising. It has an exquisite ability to sense what the person is doing, and according to preprogrammed rules, it offers assistance as needed. As the person improves over the course of therapy, the robotic device backs off the amount of assistance it's providing, leading to better function. Robotic-assisted devices are a contemporary technological method of providing the repetitive assistance that a therapist would normally provide, without the physical strain on the therapist. We know that the patients need to perform many repetitions, and these robotic devices can do it tirelessly. It's a great way to embrace emerging technology to the benefit of patients.

The duration of therapy with a patient is likely a critical element in achieving good results. We typically provide 18 to 36 sessions over 6 to 12 weeks, three times a week. We know that for a single session in the upper extremities, a thousand repetitions will last around an hour. That means we can get in up to 36,000 repetitions. Just like practicing a tennis serve or a swimming stroke, you need to do many repetitions. You can't simply do a few repetitions or a couple of sessions for the adaptive plasticity in the brain to actually take hold. It has to be done over a long time for durable effects.

What kind of results can people expect from robot therapy? If we take people a year after their stroke, people who have regained some function but still have some residual hemiparesis, and we engage them with the robots we use in our clinic for 36 sessions, then we expect to see change well over and above what people think is clinically meaningful on average. That said, some patients don't respond so well, and others respond well beyond that. We're trying to understand which people are responding and which are not responding and why. We're also trying to do more robust therapy by adding other treatments on top of the robot therapy, such as brain stimulation or plasticity-enhancing medication. Using this paradigm, we do see clinically meaningful effects across a whole group of subjects.

A lot of hospitals haven't embraced this technology yet, mainly because of a combination of the expense, the practicalities of training the staff, the staff's personal preference for therapies, and perhaps the efficacy data. There are a number of larger academic hospitals that have started to use this technology and see the benefits for the patients and the cost savings. As for insurance covering this type of treatment, it's not a therapy that is billed separately, but just another tool a therapist can use during a normal therapy session.

Not all robots are the same, just as not all medications are the same. They're really quite different and come in all shapes and sizes. Some are exoskeletons that look like an Iron Man suit, while others are small and bolted onto another device. In stroke recovery, we want to get people using as much of their residual biology as possible to get their muscular systems back online, instead of using full robotic suits that do things for them. There are both cardiovascular health benefits and psychological benefits to improving your own body.

There are certain things that distinguish robotic therapy devices from other kinds of exercise equipment. A robotic therapy device must have a mode that can provide assistance, and it must interact with the patient, adapting the assistance according to the abilities of the patient. If it doesn't do those two things, it isn't truly a robotic therapy device.

They're a relatively new technology, so we're still trying to understand what the key components are and what will work best. Something that's proven with one particular robot may not transfer to another robot. Something that's proven in the upper limb may not transfer to gait training because the motion of controlling the hand is different from walking. We need to look carefully at what the robotic devices are and what they do, and which ones have actually been tested on which patients. In general, the upper extremities—the arm and hand function—have been studied much better, so there's more evidence supporting robotics there. The lower extremities and gait training are arguably equally or more important, but there's a bit less data to support the use of robotics there. Both are very promising.

How much benefit we can expect, which robots are best, and which are best for which patients really depends on a couple of things: one is the patient's pathology and stage of recovery; the second is the goals of the patient. People have a finite amount of time, and they're trying to live their lives—they can't spend 100 percent of their time doing therapy. Some might be more interested in improving hand and arm function than improving gait training, and vice versa. It depends on what the person's goals are. As for the patient, a good candidate would be somebody who's not completely paralyzed—somebody with a small amount of voluntary movement.

98. What do you mean by "brain stimulation"?

Dr. Roth: There's a lot of interest and a lot of activity right now in something called *neuromodulation*, which basically is stimulation of the brain. There's *transcranial magnetic stimulation* (TMS), applying a magnetic field to the brain, and also *electrical stimulation*, applying electric current directly to the area around the brain injury or to the other side of the brain. Both are noninvasive, stimulating the outside of the skull or scalp. What's been really interesting is seeing that combining the stimulation with exercise may actually result in improvement in brain function. It's not used clinically yet for day-to-day practice, but there are lots of studies and many centers that are experimenting with this, and I expect at some point soon it will be used everywhere.

Dr. Page: We use brain stimulation at our lab. The idea of applying an electrical current to the brain has been around for quite a while. With TMS, what we're essentially doing is applying a magnetized electric coil to the scalp of the patient. Underneath the scalp is the brain that has had a stroke. Depending on where we apply the current, we can affect the part of the brain that controls walking, hand motion, or speech production. Depending on where we place the coil, we can either facilitate or inhibit those areas of the brain, making more or less activity happen in those regions.

Now the questions become, how much current we should use, how should we structure the practice that goes with that brain stimulation, and which side of the brain should we target (the side that has the lesion versus the side that doesn't, or both sides at the same time?).

What we do know is that it has an effect; there's very good evidence suggesting that it seems to speed the process of recovery after a stroke, and we're pretty sure what the mechanisms are. Unfortunately, it's not something that is widely used in rehabilitation at this point because it's not FDA approved for stroke right now. At the moment, brain stimulation is approved only for depression. We know it's safe. The only side effect is seizures; they're rare, but they do happen. We're very concerned with safety in applying something to the brain, so we use established screening criteria before using it.

Another type of brain stimulation is *transcranial direct current stimulation* (tDCS). tDCS is safer than TMS because we're applying a less focal and less powerful current to the brain. The procedures are basically the same. We're using electrodes and a low-level stimulator instead of a big coil. The amount of stimulation is much lower in tDCS, so it's even safer.

A Status Report on Brain Stimulation from Dr. Mike

Transcranial magnetic stimulation, or TMS, is one form of brain stimulation. There are several different types: single-pulse TMS, repetitive TMS (rTMS), deep TMS (dTMS), and navigated TMS (nTMS). TMS is currently FDA approved for the treatment of depression, but clinical trials suggest that TMS may also act as an effective part of stroke recovery treatment by stimulating growth in brain cells. These stimulation devices are currently used to help stroke survivors make faster gains in their recoveries at university hospitals conducting research. Combining TMS with other standard therapies may help patients regain speech and movement. Nexstim is a company focusing their research on TMS and stroke recovery. Their Contrastim Stroke Study found that people who received TMS combined with occupational therapy made more gains than patients receiving occupational therapy alone. After these promising results, Nexstim conducted a trial at 12 of the top rehabilitation sites in the United States.

A phase-three trial found no safety concerns in the patients enrolled in the trial.

While TMS is currently considered off-label for stroke recovery, doctors who already use it in their practices to treat depression may be willing to use these devices to help stroke survivors. Before deciding to undergo TMS, however, patients should talk to their doctors to learn the risks and benefits of this treatment.

While legal, off-label uses are not covered by health insurance. If you're paying out of pocket, a course of TMS is expensive, costing several thousand dollars. Health insurance *does* sometimes cover TMS if it is being used to treat depression that has not responded to antidepressants, so this is an affordable option for stroke survivors who are also experiencing depression. Since up to one-third of stroke survivors experience depression, this can be a worthwhile, drug-free alternative to prescription antidepressants.

As of 2016 there are four TMS devices that are FDA approved for depression: Neuronetics' NeuroStar TMS Therapy System, MagVenture's MagVita TMS Therapy, Magstim's Rapid^2 Therapy System, and Brainsway's Deep TMS. To find a provider near you, check their websites: www.NeuroStar.com, www.MagVenture.com, www.Magstim.com, and www.Brainsway.com.

Nexstim's Navigated Brain Therapy (NBT) System treats stroke and is based on TMS technology. Initial studies of this TMS combined with therapy show a twofold improvement when compared to therapy alone. Nexstim is preparing to seek FDA clearance for using the NBT System in stroke rehabilitation. You can follow updates on the status of the Nexstim NBT System on their website at www.Nexstim.com.

Transcranial direct current stimulation, or tDCS, is another form of brain stimulation being researched. Like TMS, tDCS is not currently FDA approved for the treatment of stroke rehabilitation. However, there are doctors who may be willing to use the device off-label to treat stroke survivors. But remember: since it's not FDA approved, it won't be covered by insurance. Again, tDCS would have to be combined with physical, occupational, and speech therapy to maximize effectiveness. Stay away from tDCS devices being sold on the Internet for home use. They could potentially be dangerous for a stroke survivor as a tDCS device must be specialized to meet the unique needs of a stroke survivor.

Dr. Roth: There's intriguing research on what's called *brain-computer interface*. This is when you implant electrodes in the brain, and then the electrodes sense what the brain's thinking and convert that into the movements of a computer or prosthetic device. The electrodes are there to sense the electricity of the brain instead of stimulate it. The brain-computer interface is still very experimental, mostly because it requires neurosurgery to implant the electrodes. Now there's some research looking at placing electrodes on the surface of the scalp instead, using what looks like a bathing cap with electrodes all over it. The person will wear those electrodes to let the computer read the brain waves and be able to act. Keep in mind that the brain waves are not read very clearly because you've got the whole scalp to go through. It's a very interesting approach, but we're still a ways away from using it.

99. What's the scoop with stem cell therapy?

Dr. Chiu: A very exciting area of research is in *stem cell therapy*, or cellular therapy. These treatments are now in randomized, controlled clinical trials, and so far the results are promising. The stem cell therapies we're investigating now may modify the inflammatory reaction that occurs in an acute stroke, as well as enhance *neurogenesis* and *angiogenesis* (the development of new brain cells and blood vessels) through a growth-factor effect.

Dr. Carmichael: Stem cell therapies really look hopeful for the stroke recovery field. It's a pregnant moment because the science of neurorepair in the brain is reaching a maturation point. We have strong candidates for drugs that might promote recovery. It's going to take 5 to 10 years, but at least we're there in the laboratory stage. The ability to enhance neuroplasticity with a cellular therapeutic is being seen in the preclinical studies of the rodent models of stroke, promoting dramatic recovery. Now we're in the phase of understanding why that occurs and how we might translate it to humans. We understand stem cell biology more, and we're starting to understand how to work with stem cells to make them applicable to human brain diseases. In some cases we're now in phase-two clinical trials that might provide a therapeutic option. It's a pretty dramatic scientific time.

When people say "stem cells," they mean a lot of different things. The best clinical trials to date that have shown recovery have been early phase-one trials. They were looking to see if stem cell therapy was safe, but there were some really surprising examples of people with chronic stroke who got dramatically better. Now these treatments are moving into phase two. These treatments involved direct cell injections into the brain through a very small hole in the skull. Stem cells are a big field, there are a lot of therapies being tested, and we're still a ways from a clinically validated approach, but it's very promising.

The most important thing to realize is that we are still about five to seven years away from a clinically tested and validated stem cell therapy. In Southern California a lot of patients will go to Mexico to get cell injections and therapies that are not clinically validated. It's not always known what is being done to the patient—in some cases it causes harm—and it always costs a lot. These offshore therapeutics are a concerning element in the field. We must be patient. There's a real risk of patients falling prey to people who are not physicians but really business entrepreneurs who are promoting these approaches.

"We all want to be better instantly. There is no simple cure for stroke, so we have to adapt for now. I use a lot of assistive technology to help me adapt to my language problems and being

one-handed. It took me a long time to accept that I am not going to recover 100 percent, but I can still live the life I want. I've already exceeded all expectations in my hard-fought recovery journey, and new treatments like stem cells make me hopeful that I'll be taking my recovery to the next level someday soon." — David

A Tip from Dr. Mike

"One of the most toxic feelings to human beings is hopelessness, so I'm incredibly excited that there's so much progress in the world of stroke recovery to help us all feel hopeful. When I stumbled across the results of the first major study of stem cell therapy for stroke survivors, I thought, "Wow! How can I get this for David?" My family and I already have hope because we see the man David has become and the progress he's made. Now it appears there is new, game-changing research that gives us even more hope. So today, use all the therapies and treatments that are readily available along with the simple lifestyle changes in diet and exercise that we know work. Tomorrow, you can look forward to the dawn of a new era of treatment. In all likelihood, combination therapy, which combines the tried-and-true therapies we have now with cutting-edge treatments like stem cell therapy, will be the answer so many stroke survivors are now seeking."

The Promise of Stem Cell Therapy from Dr. Mike

Clinical trials using stem cells in stroke survivors started in 2005, and the results of the trials have exceeded expectations. There are four questions researchers are seeking to answer through these trials: Is it safe? Does it work? Is it more effective than existing therapies? What are the long-term results and side effects, if any? With the promising results of recent studies, it appears stem cell therapy could be a widely available and incredibly effective treatment for stroke survivors in the next 5 to 10 years. Research using stem cells in stroke rehabilitation is progressing rapidly, so consult reputable sources and your doctors to stay informed about the latest updates. Here is a glimpse of what recent stem cell studies have found:

- In one study, stem cells were safely infused into the brain through the carotid artery when given two weeks after a stroke. There were no harmful effects in any patients in the trial after a year of stem cell injections. Co-principal investigator of this study Dileep R. Yavagal, MD, said, "The conclusions of our research prove that stem cells are safe when given through the carotid artery with a small catheter." Ralph L. Sacco, MD, chief of neurology service at Jackson Memorial Hospital, which was one of the sites of this study, said, "This study opens the door to future clinical trials that will explore new methods of repairing damage to the brain with cell-based therapies. Stroke researchers now know that stem cells can be used safely and efficiently without compromising the health of the patient. We have more work to do in this promising area to improve the outcomes of our stroke patients."

- Following the success of that study, stem cells were safely infused directly into the brains of stroke survivors by using a procedure that required just one night in the hospital. The patients in this study had a stroke between six months and three years prior to treatment. Gary Steinberg, MD, who led the trial, said, "It was designed primarily to test the procedure's safety. But patients improved by several standard measures. . . . Their ability to move around has recovered visibly. That's unprecedented.

. . . Some patients couldn't walk. Others couldn't move their arm. This wasn't just 'They couldn't move their thumb, and now they can.' Patients who were in wheelchairs are walking now. We know these cells don't survive for more than a month or so in the brain, yet we see that patients' recovery is sustained for greater than one year and, in some cases now, more than two years. Older people tend not to respond to treatment as well, but here we see 70-year-olds recovering substantially. . . . We thought those brain circuits were dead. And we've learned that they're not." As of June 2016, these researchers are seeking to enroll subjects in a multi-center phase-2b trial.

- Stem cell therapy research in stroke survivors is now taking place around the world. In November 2015 the first stem cell injection in a 66-year-old stroke survivor in England was used to help the woman regain use of her arm. Soon, stem cell therapy may be available to stroke survivors in the United States and abroad.

• • • • •

Takeaway Points:

The future of stroke recovery is very bright. In the next few years and decades, we will be seeing many new treatments that will have powerful results when combined. Be on the lookout for these advances:

- Better assistive technology to help you do the things you can't

- Robotic therapy that provides assistance as it adapts to your abilities

- Electromagnetic stimulation that activates or inhibits certain parts of the brain

- Stem cell therapeutics that help the brain create new connections or heal faster

All these advances must undergo extensive research and testing for safety and efficacy. Be careful of people selling unapproved treatments. Until new treatments are approved for stroke, focus on the therapy and principles that are proven to work.

CHAPTER 14

A LAST WORD
OF ADVICE

100. What is the one message—one piece of advice—that you would give all stroke survivors?

Dr. Carmichael: Be hopeful and active. The core element there is *hope*. With stroke it's a constant effort, and it certainly takes a lot of attention, but there's hope for community integration, interaction with loved ones, and recovery of function that never really goes away.

Dr. Chiu: The field of stroke recovery is very exciting right now. Apart from the research and investigational treatments, standard *therapy works* to promote recovery and can go on even more than a year after a stroke. It can continue. Don't underestimate that.

Dr. Edwards: The brain has the capability of reorganizing and adapting for improved function, but it's not a passive process. It requires meaningful daily effort from the individual, just like learning an instrument. If you want to improve, you have to seek guidance, be active, and *never give up*.

Dr. Gillen: You are ultimately responsible for your own recovery, improvement, and care. You can't just sit and wait for the next therapy session to happen and not do anything in between. You need to *take* *control* of your rehabilitation in terms of doing independent practice and maximizing your participation in everyday life. Don't become sedentary or stop engaging in life—you're going to get out as much as you put in.

Dr. Hinckley: Finding a *balance* in this new life of living with stroke is really critical. You don't have to carry the whole burden yourself. In fact if you do, it's likely to be detrimental, so it's important to find good ways of coping.

Dr. Hinkle: Be a great *advocate*. Don't be afraid to ask hard questions or offend people. Speak up for yourself (or your loved one). Become a pain in the neck to get what you need.

Dr. Holland: Recovery can go on and on for many years following a stroke. It's important that people who have had a stroke and their families don't give up hope and continue to *be optimistic* and resilient about the ultimate long-term recovery.

Dr. Monroe: You have to decide whether you want to be your disability or you want to *be yourself*. Don't forget who you are. Try new things even though you might be afraid or think you can't do them. Practice your skills in playful settings where if you don't succeed it's not going to cause you significant problems, and focus on the good in your life.

Dr. Page: Your target is not arm movement, walking faster, or speaking better; those are all things that are nice to happen, but your target is the brain and *changing the brain*. If you change the brain, then all those other things are going to happen. We change the brain through thousands and thousands and thousands of attempts—through practice. That's how the brain learns, and that's how the brain rewires.

Dr. Ploughman: Take those first six months to really *drive plasticity* as much as you can by capitalizing on everything around you. If you have physiotherapists, occupational therapists, and speech-language pathologists, have them map out activities for you to do. Beyond the hour or so you spend with them a couple of times a week, take more time to work during those six months when plasticity is at its highest.

Dr. Roth: It's important to always keep in mind how essential your *determination* is. Stay motivated, stay active, and stay engaged. Do everything you can to advocate for yourself, to be treated with respect and dignity, to be communicated with and educated, and to be taken seriously.

Dr. Stoykov: You have to *be motivated* if you want to get better. You can't just expect that going to therapy a few hours a week or going to a research study is going to result in a big recovery. You need to do so many hours a day. You have to be doing things at home. You have to keep moving.

Ms. Thompson: I am constantly inspired by the stroke survivors that I work with—seeing their attitude and drive to live life to the fullest and be the best they can be. I want to encourage people to remember to have fun and *enjoy life* as much as possible.

Dr. Woodward: You're not alone. Other people have experienced this, and you can learn from those experiences—don't shut people out. Know that recovery is a long-term process. You're in it for the long haul. *Find support* to help you deal with the ups and downs, and try not to let the downs completely overcome you.

And from Dr. Mike and David

You've reached the end of the book, but your journey has just begun. We hope this text has provided you with both information and inspiration. Whoever you are and wherever you on this path, the time has come for action. There's no stop sign on this road to recovery. It's time for you to go and heal your broken brain. We dedicate this book to all stroke survivors and their advocates.

APPENDIX A: RESOURCES
FOR YOUR RECOVERY

Stroke Information

When searching the web for information on stroke, it's important to look for reputable sources that are intended for survivors and
families. These organizations provide current and accurate information you can trust:

American Stroke Association: strokeassociation.org
The leading nonprofit organization in the United States dedicated
to prevention, diagnosis, and treatment to save lives from stroke.

Heart & Stroke Foundation: heartandstroke.com
Go to Health Information > Stroke for excellent informational
resources on all aspects of stroke and stroke recovery from this trusted
Canadian organization. Click on Free Publications to download *Your
Stroke Journey: A guide for people living with stroke*, a 110-page book.

National Stroke Association: stroke.org
A nonprofit U.S.-based organization that provides free stroke education and programs to stroke survivors, caregivers, and the health-
care community to reduce the incidence and impact of stroke.

Stroke Association: stroke.org.uk

This British stroke association has an incredible library of documents on stroke recovery that are free to download. Go to Finding Support > Publications for a complete list you can filter by theme.

Stroke Engine: strokengine.ca

Click on Interventions to find out which treatments have good research evidence behind them. Written for both families and clinicians, this site helps you understand best practices in stroke recovery.

Stroke Magazines

Stroke Connection: strokeconnection.org

This free digital magazine about stroke comes out four times a year and is published by the American Stroke Association. It is filled with stories of stroke survivors, recovery, and hope. You can read the current and past issues online anytime. Subscribe by e-mail so you know when a new issue comes out.

StrokeSmart: strokesmart.org

A free magazine for stroke survivors published by the National Stroke Association. Print and digital subscriptions are available, along with articles on the website. Stories focus on poststroke living, recovery, and resources for stroke survivors.

Finding Local Services

Stroke-certified hospitals: strokecenter.org/trials/centers/

Find your nearest stroke-certified hospital or rehabilitation center by using this user-friendly search tool. To download the full list of stroke-certified hospitals, go to qualitycheck.org; then select Stroke Certification.

Clinical research trials: clinicaltrials.gov

Search this database of all registered human clinical trials around the world. Look for stroke studies in your area to see if you may qualify. You may not get the experimental treatment, and even if you do, it may not work, but you are playing an important role in advancing research by participating.

One-Handed Living

While we know it's best to always try to use both hands, there are many stroke survivors who live with functional use of just one hand. Your occupational therapist can help you find ways to do everyday activities with one hand by using **special techniques** (like one-handed shoe tying) and adaptive equipment, as well as ways to keep using your affected hand as much as possible. Being one-handed is not an excuse to stop you from being as independent as you want to be.

The Internet is full of **products specific to one-handed living**: cutting boards, can openers, pepper grinders, dressing aids, nail clippers, hair-dryer holders, lipped plates, rocker knives, card holders, book stands, toothpaste dispensers, elastic shoelaces, hair ties, bra fasteners, and more. Dycem's nonslip film acts as a flat suction cup you can place under plates, paper, or anything that slides. A lower-cost alternative is to cut squares from a roll of nonadhesive padded shelf liner. A foam tube can make a spoon or pencil easier to hold in your affected hand, and a few stainless steel nails in a cutting board can hold vegetables while you slice. Be creative—necessity is the mother of invention.

Look for **everyday tools** that make life easier for everyone. Bluetooth devices can free up your hands, while electronic readers eliminate the need to hold a book open. Terry-cloth bathrobes double as towels, and disposable flossers make it easier to clean your teeth. Adaptive equipment intended for people with arthritis or shoulder surgery, amputees, and the elderly are often good for stroke survivors too. There are even recipes written for people cooking with one hand, such as parents who are carrying a baby in one arm while making dinner. If there's something you're struggling to do, **search to find a solution** online, look on YouTube, or ask your stroke support group. You're not the only one living with one good arm!

One-Handed in a Two-Handed World: Your Complete Guide to Managing Single-Handedly is an older book by Tommye-Karen Mayer with insights on every aspect of daily life for people using only one hand. It's out of print now, but if you can find a copy, it may be helpful if you're struggling to find solutions or looking for ways to promote independence.

Further Reading on Cognition

There are a few books about people with cognitive or perceptual problems after brain damage that may help you better understand what it's like. *The Man Who Mistook His Wife for a Hat* is a book by Oliver Sacks that features stories of many different neurological phenomena including many from damage to the right hemisphere of the brain. *Left Neglected* by Lisa Genova deals with a woman with left neglect after a brain injury.

Dr. Mike's book *The Brain Fog Fix* addresses memory, mood, and proven brain health strategies that are effective for all people— whether their brains are affected by a stroke or the simple wear and tear of daily life.

Aphasia

Aphasia Recovery Connection's Guide to Living with Aphasia by Amanda P. Anderson, MS, CCC-SLP, and Carol Dow-Richards is an indispensable book for families dealing with loss of language after a stroke. Available on Amazon.com

The National Aphasia Association (aphasia.org) provides information about aphasia and lists support groups and programs across the United States.

AphasiaAccess (aphasiaaccess.org/program-roster) also lists aphasia centers that use the *life participation approach to aphasia* (LPAA).

Aphasia Recovery Connection (aphasiarc.org) is an aphasia support group that anyone can access via Facebook. They offer online support groups for stroke survivors and caregivers, events like cruises with conferences specifically for people with aphasia and their families, and an Aphasia University Boot Camp in Las Vegas, a 28-day educational and social program. To learn more, go to page 201.

The Aphasia Institute (aphasia.ca) in Toronto offers training in the formal principles of Supported Conversation for Adults with Aphasia (SCA), as well as pictograph-filled books to help people with aphasia communicate with medical professionals or discuss complex topics.

The Aphasia Software Finder (aphasiasoftwarefinder.org) lists all the aphasia computer programs and apps for therapy.

Tactus Therapy (tactustherapy.com) offers affordable therapy apps and resources for stroke survivors with aphasia. Free *Lite* apps are available to try on Apple and Android touch-screen devices. The blog has helpful articles about speech therapy and using technology. To learn more, go to page 199.

YouTube has many videos about aphasia: youtube.com/user/aphasia channel/playlists. Learn more about aphasia, see therapy in action, and watch stroke survivors progress year after year as they recover.

Stroke Support Groups

In-Person Groups

Your local stroke hospital or rehab center should be able to point you to stroke support groups in your area. The meetings are often held in hospitals, libraries, or community centers. Visit the websites for the stroke organizations listed in the beginning of this appendix to search for support groups in your area. If you can't find one, consider starting one.

Online Groups

There are many groups on Facebook that provide a forum to connect stroke survivors and caregivers. Here are a few of the most popular groups with thousands of members:

- Stroke Survivors: facebook.com/groups/573759576077398/

- Young Stroke Survivors: facebook.com/groups/5326941831/

- Aphasia Recovery Connection: facebook.com/groups/Aphasia.Recovery.Connection/

- Stroke Caregivers: facebook.com/groups/215998465086406/

Assistance Programs

211

Dial 211 or visit 211.org for free, confidential help with finding local resources for health and human services during a personal crisis. It is funded by the United Way and available in North America. It can help you find assistance with housing, food, employment, health care, support groups, addiction, and abuse.

There are several in-home and out-of-home respite care services available. Learn more about the Administration on Aging's National Family Caregiver Support Program and find resources at aoa.acl.gov. There you will find a link to two referral sources for respite care in your area:

- The Eldercare Locator is a public service of the Administration on Aging. Information can be found online at eldercare.gov or by phone at 1-800-677-1116.

- ARCH National Respite Network and Resource Center has a local directory of respite providers at https://archrespite.org/respitelocator.

If a stroke survivor is also a veteran, family members can call the VA Caregiver Support line at 1-855-260-3274 or visit them online at caregiver.va.gov.

ABOUT TACTUS THERAPY

Tactus Therapy offers a variety of evidence-based apps and resources for stroke survivors and their families. These apps are available for you to enhance your recovery at home by *maximizing neuroplasticity* with repeated practice. Tactus Therapy believes that you should have access to affordable professional tools you can use anytime, anywhere, for unrestricted therapy. That's why these apps, designed by a speech-language pathologist, are made just for you— the adult stroke survivor—to give you a personalized experience that puts you in control of your recovery.

All these touch-screen apps have free Lite versions that you can try for yourself or show to your therapist for personalized recommendations. Download them onto your phone or tablet from the App Store or Google Play.

- **Language Therapy 4-in-1** targets speaking, understanding, reading, and writing for those with moderate-to-severe aphasia. An independent study shows that using this app just 20 minutes a day can make a significant improvement in language skills for people with chronic aphasia.

- **Advanced Naming Therapy** and **Advanced Comprehension Therapy** expand on the Language Therapy skills to challenge you as you improve.

- **Apraxia Therapy** uses powerful video modeling to help people with aphasia to speak.

- **Conversation Therapy** provides topics to discuss with a partner so you can both work on your communication strategies.

- **Category Therapy, Number Therapy,** and **Question Therapy 2-in-1** help with speaking and understanding specific types of language with a variety of activities.

- **Visual Attention Therapy** helps people with left neglect—a perceptual problem common after stroke—to scan the screen visually.

Visit tactustherapy.com for more information on each app and to learn how apps can enhance your recovery. Sign up for the free newsletter and follow the blog for engaging stories, helpful education, and exciting developments in speech therapy for stroke recovery.

"While I've downloaded quite a number of iPad applications to assist with my husband's stroke recovery, the Tactus Therapy apps are the only ones he wants to use. The ease of the user interface is simple enough for him to use the apps on his own. He loves to watch his score as he gets the answers correct and is so proud of his progress. All of his doctors are amazed at his progress and say his level of recovery with his speech is nothing short of miraculous." —Debra W., wife of a stroke survivor

ABOUT APHASIA RECOVERY CONNECTION

Aphasia Recovery Connection (ARC) is a nonprofit organization working to help end the isolation of aphasia. They host several online Facebook groups to connect people with aphasia, as well as high-quality events such as Aphasia Learning @ Sea cruises and Aphasia University Boot Camp. ARC creates a community that really understands aphasia, and it is open to all people with aphasia, their family members, their care partners, and professionals.

ARC was started after David Dow met another young stroke survivor. Christine Huggins was just 26 when she had a stroke, bringing her career as an attorney to a premature end. Christine and David, assisted by their mothers, Kim and Carol, set out to make a difference by giving others with aphasia and their caregivers a means to connect and help each other.

Aphasia Recovery Connection offers a place to find motivation, inspiration, and education—as well as a place to ask questions of other families or of speech therapists. After a stroke, friends either disappear or don't call as often. People with aphasia and their caregivers do not always have access to speech therapy or other resources. Often people with aphasia are released from the hospital once their immediate health-care needs are met, but they're left with so many unanswered questions.

Aphasia Recovery Connection provides a platform and resources for people with aphasia and their caregivers to connect with others who truly understand what they are going through. Through Facebook groups online, aphasia cruises at sea, and boot camps in Las

Vegas—they share stories, advice, tips, tools, and resources and help each other navigate the road to recovery.

ARC's mission is to deliver compassionate support services to improve the quality of life for people recovering from aphasia and their families and friends. We are committed to helping to end the isolation that aphasia brings. We embody the values of collaboration, compassion, dignity, and acceptance.

See what ARC has to offer you and your family. Connect with us!

Website: aphasiarc.org
E-mail: arcteam@aphasiarecoveryconnection.org
Facebook: facebook.com/aphasiaARC/

APPENDIX B: MEET THE EXPERTS

Dr. S. Thomas Carmichael, MD, PhD, is a neurologist and neuroscientist at UCLA. Dr. Carmichael is a professor of neurology and co-director of the UCLA Broad Stem Cell Research Center, with clinical interests in stroke and neurorehabilitation and how the brain repairs from injury. Dr. Carmichael's laboratory studies the mechanisms of brain repair and functional recovery after stroke along with stem cell treatments. He is an attending physician in the neuro-rehabilitation and stroke clinical programs at UCLA.

Dr. David Chiu, MD, is the medical director of the Houston Methodist Eddy Scurlock Stroke Center in Houston, Texas, and a neurologist at the Houston Methodist Neurological Institute. He serves on the board of directors for the American Heart Association. He is also a reviewer for the journal *Stroke* and the *Journal of Neurology, Neurosurgery & Psychiatry*. Dr. Chiu is a professor of clinical neurology at Cornell University. He received his MD from Yale University. Dr. Chiu's research interests lie in extending the time and quality of life for stroke patients, acute stroke treatment, and stroke prevention in those who have experienced TIA and stroke.

Dr. Dylan Edwards, PhD, PT, is the director of the Noninvasive Brain Stimulation and Human Motor Control Laboratory at the Burke Rehabilitation Hospital in New York. Dr. Edwards is a neuroscientist and a physical therapist with expertise in motor recovery through robotic neurorehabilitation and brain electrical stimulation. He is accelerating the advancement of cutting-edge technological neurorehabilitation therapies to promote long-lasting improvements for impairments caused by neurological injuries.

Dr. Glen Gillen, EdD, OTR, is an associate professor of rehabilitation and regenerative medicine in occupational therapy at Columbia University. He has authored more than 70 publications, including textbooks, chapters, and peer-reviewed research and serves on the editorial boards for several journals related to physical medicine and rehabilitation. Dr. Gillen is best known for his textbooks *Stroke Rehabilitation: A Function-Based Approach,* now in its fourth edition, and *Cognitive and Perceptual Rehabilitation: Optimizing Function.* Dr. Gillen is an award-winning occupational therapist specializing in neurorehabilitation, with an active clinical caseload in acute care and inpatient rehabilitation.

Dr. Jacqueline J. Hinckley, PhD, CCC-SLP, is an associate professor emeritus of speech-language pathology at the University of South Florida. She currently serves as executive director for Voices of Hope for Aphasia. She is an experienced consultant, trainer, presenter, researcher, and clinician focused on bringing evidence-supported interventions to stroke and brain injury rehabilitation.

Dr. Janice L. Hinkle, PhD, CNRN, is the president of the American Association of Neuroscience Nurses and editor in chief of the *Journal of Nursing Measurement.* She is also a fellow at Villanova University. She has decades of experience as a clinical nurse specialist and earned her PhD in nursing from the University of Pennsylvania.

Dr. Audrey Holland, PhD, CCC-SLP, is a world-renowned aphasia researcher and advocate. She is the Regents' professor emeritus of speech, language, and hearing sciences at the University of Arizona and has served on the advisory council for the U.S. National Institute on Deafness and other Communication Disorders. Dr. Holland has been awarded several of the highest honors from speech-language pathology and aphasia professional associations. She has published and edited hundreds of research articles, book chapters, and reviews, in addition to developing several communication assessments.

Dr. Janice Elich Monroe, PhD, CTRS, is an associate professor and chair of the Department of Recreation and Leisure Studies at Ithaca College in New York. Her research and scholarly interests include contemplative education and mindfulness, the use of multisensory environments in the treatment of individuals with disabilities, and the role of leisure in society. Dr. Monroe serves as the recreation therapy clinical supervisor at the Center for Life Skills, an interdisciplinary program tailored to meet the individual needs of adults who have experienced a stroke or other neurological impairment.

Dr. Stephen Page, PhD, OTR, is an associate professor of occupational therapy at The Ohio State University. A prolific researcher, writer, and speaker, he leads the B.R.A.I.N. Lab to develop and test approaches that increase function and independence after stroke and other neurological diseases. Dr. Page believes in translating scientific research into real-life practice, organizing neurorehabilitation conferences for clinicians, and mentoring students while maintaining his clinical practice as an OT in the community. He has co-developed the Certified Stroke Rehabilitation Specialist program for occupational and physical therapists to become stroke-certified clinicians. Dr. Page is a fellow of both the American Heart Association and the American Congress of Rehabilitation Medicine.

Dr. Michelle Ploughman, PhD, PT, is an assistant professor in physical medicine and rehabilitation at Memorial University in Canada. She is a physical therapist and neuroscientist and a recognized expert in neuroplasticity and neurorehabilitation in stroke and multiple sclerosis. Her research focuses on the effects of aerobic exercise, intensive training paradigms, and lifestyle habits on the brain challenged by injury, disease, and aging. Dr. Ploughman is a Canada Research Chair in neuroplasticity, neurorehabilitation, and brain recovery. Dr. Ploughman continues to practice as a neurological physiotherapist in St. John's, Newfoundland.

Dr. Elliot J. Roth, MD, is a professor and chairman of the Department of Physical Medicine and Rehabilitation at Northwestern University Feinberg School of Medicine, chairman of the Department of Rehabilitation Medicine at Northwestern Memorial Hospital, and medical director of the Patient Recovery Unit at the Rehabilitation Institute of Chicago. Dr. Roth specializes in the rehabilitation of patients with stroke, traumatic brain injury, spinal cord injury, and other disabling conditions. His research and academic interests are in the areas of novel methods to enhance recovery, improve functional outcomes, and prevent associated medical conditions for people with disabling conditions.

Dr. Mary Ellen Stoykov, PhD, OT, is an assistant professor of occupational therapy at Rush University in Chicago. She has many years of clinical experience working as an occupational therapist in chronic pain, stroke, and traumatic brain injury. Additionally, Dr. Stoykov is a researcher in the area of poststroke upper-limb hemiparesis and has served as a research occupational therapist at the Rehabilitation Institute of Chicago.

Sarah Thompson, MM, MT-BC, CBIS, is an award-winning and board-certified music therapist and brain injury specialist. She is a fellow in neurological music therapy and has served as adjunct faculty for the music therapy program at Colorado State University. She runs the Rehabilitative Rhythms music therapy clinic serving the Denver area.

Dr. Amanda Toler Woodward, PhD, is an associate professor in the School of Social Work at Michigan State University. She is currently a co-investigator on the Michigan Stroke Transitions Trial, which looks at improving care transitions for acute stroke patients through a patient-centered, home-based case management program.

INDEX

A

Academic medical centers, 92–93

Activities. *See* Games; Recreational therapy

Acupuncture, 113–114

Acute stage of recovery, 25

Adaptive strategies, 88–89

Advice, last words of, 187–189

Advice, other. *See* David, thoughts on topics; *specific names of professionals*; *specific topics*

Aerobic training, 41, 42, 112, 118

African Americans, stroke risk, 8

Age, recovery and, 27

Age, stroke risk and, 4, 8–9

Alcohol, 7, 10, 111

Alzheimer's disease. *See* Dementia

Ankle-foot orthosis (AFO), 44

Anticoagulant medications, 11, 22

Aphasia. *See also* Communication, recovering
about: takeaway points, 83
apraxia and, 70
communication tips, 75–79
decision-making and, 82
defined, 70
experience example, 71
family helping with recovery, 74–75
helping with words or not, 77–78
intelligence, cognitive abilities and, 70–71, 75
mental health and, 146–147
resources (additional), 194–195
supported communication and, 74–75
support groups/information, 78–79, 194–196
technology helping with, 79–82
terminal uniqueness caution, 74
types of, 71
view of what recovery looks like with, 72
watching TV and, 82

Aphasia Recovery Connection, xv, xx, 74, 80, 81, 168, 195, 196, 201–202

Aphasia Recovery Connection's Guide to Living with Aphasia (Anderson), 194

Apps
calculator, 67
calendar, 66
camera, 66
clock, 66
for communication, 80–81
contacts, 66
finding and using, 79–80, 81, 147, 195
finding friends, 67
health tracking, 67
helping with aphasia, 80
maps, 66
meditation, 147
notes and reminders, 67
smartphone, 65–67
Tactus Therapy, xii–xiii, 81, 195, 199–200
for tracking exercise, 55, 79
voice memos, 67

Apraxia, 70

Arm and hand, recovering, 49–57
about: overview of, 49; takeaway points, 57
challenges unique to, 49–50
connection between brain and, 50
constraint-induced movement therapy (CIMT) and, xi–xii, 52–54
flapper for bilateral priming, 55
getting hands working, 50–51
keeping arm moving to decrease pain, 50
learned nonuse and, 51
making one-handed life easier, 56–57, 193–194
mirror therapy, 54
myoelectric device for, 56
sensory feedback and, 50
technology helping with, 54–56
time frame for, 51

Assistance programs, 196–197

Assistive technology, 174, 181–182

Atrial fibrillation, 11, 113

ACKNOWLEDGMENTS

Special thanks to:
Carol Dow-Richards and Laura Gray

ABOUT THE AUTHORS

Dr. Mike Dow, PsyD, is a psychotherapist, author, and host of health-oriented TV and radio shows. Informed by his own personal experiences, Dr. Mike believes in the brain's ability to heal itself. Dr. Mike's first book, *Diet Rehab*, is now available in three languages. His second book, *The Brain Fog Fix*, is a *New York Times* bestseller. Dr. Mike makes regular appearances on the *Dr. Oz Show*, *The Doctors*, and *Dr. Drew On Call* and is the host of *The Dr. Mike Show* on Hay House Radio. He has hosted shows on TLC, VH1, and E! For more information, go to www.drmikedow.com.

David Dow is a childhood stroke survivor and founding member and vice president of the Aphasia Recovery Connection, an online aphasia support group that hosts events around the country. He has published his story in *Brain Attack: My Journey of Recovery from Stroke and Aphasia*. He frequently presents to audiences of speech-language pathologists and stroke survivors to share his experience.

Megan Sutton, MS, CCC-SLP, is an award-winning speech-language pathologist and expert in using technology for communication in stroke rehabilitation. She has designed more than 20 evidence-based apps for adult-focused speech-language therapy with her company Tactus Therapy Solutions. She consults with stroke and aphasia groups around the world and is a frequent writer and presenter, helping professionals and stroke survivors learn how best to incorporate technology into therapy. Megan is a graduate of Boston University and lives in Vancouver, Canada.

Hay House Titles of Related Interest

YOU CAN HEAL YOUR LIFE, the movie, starring Louise Hay & Friends
(available as a 1-DVD program and as an expanded 2-DVD set)
Watch the trailer at: www.LouiseHayMovie.com

THE SHIFT, the movie,
starring Dr. Wayne W. Dyer
(available as a 1-DVD program and as an expanded 2-DVD set)
Watch the trailer at: www.DyerMovie.com

• • • • •

The Brain Fog Fix: Reclaim Your Focus, Memory,
and Joy in Just 3 Weeks, by Dr. Mike Dow

Loving Yourself to Great Health: Thoughts & Food—the Ultimate Diet,
by Louise Hay, Ahlea Khadro, and Heather Dane

Heal Your Mind: Your Prescription for Wholeness through Medicine, Affirmations,
and Intuition, by Mona Lisa Schulz, MD, PhD,
with Louise Hay

Breaking the Habit of Being Yourself: How to Lose
Your Mind and Create a New One, by Dr. Joe Dispenza

Power Up Your Brain: The Neuroscience of Enlightenment,
by David Perlmutter, MD, FACN, and Alberto Villoldo, PhD

All of the above are available at your local bookstore,
or may be ordered by contacting Hay House (see next page).

• • • • •

We hope you enjoyed this Hay House book. If you'd like to receive our online catalog featuring additional information on Hay House books and products, or if you'd like to find out more about the Hay Foundation, please contact:

Hay House, Inc., P.O. Box 5100, Carlsbad, CA 92018-5100
(760) 431-7695 or (800) 654-5126
(760) 431-6948 (fax) or (800) 650-5115 (fax)
www.hayhouse.com® • www.hayfoundation.org

• • • • •

Published and distributed in Australia by: Hay House Australia Pty. Ltd., 18/36 Ralph St., Alexandria NSW 2015
Phone: 612-9669-4299 • *Fax:* 612-9669-4144 • www.hayhouse.com.au

Published and distributed in the United Kingdom by: Hay House UK, Ltd., Astley House, 33 Notting Hill Gate, London W11 3JQ
Phone: 44-20-3675-2450 • *Fax:* 44-20-3675-2451 • www.hayhouse.co.uk

Published and distributed in the Republic of South Africa by:
Hay House SA (Pty), Ltd., P.O. Box 990, Witkoppen 2068
info@hayhouse.co.za • www.hayhouse.co.za

Published in India by: Hay House Publishers India, Muskaan Complex, Plot No. 3, B-2, Vasant Kunj, New Delhi 110 070
Phone: 91-11-4176-1620 • *Fax:* 91-11-4176-1630 • www.hayhouse.co.in

Distributed in Canada by: Raincoast Books, 2440 Viking Way, Richmond, B.C. V6V 1N2
Phone: 1-800-663-5714 • *Fax:* 1-800-565-3770 • www.raincoast.com

• • • • •

Take Your Soul on a Vacation

Visit www.HealYourLife.com® to regroup, recharge, and reconnect with your own magnificence.
Featuring blogs, mind-body-spirit news, and life-changing wisdom from Louise Hay and friends.

Visit www.HealYourLife.com today!

Free e-newsletters from Hay House, the Ultimate Resource for Inspiration

Be the first to know about Hay House's dollar deals, free downloads, special offers, affirmation cards, giveaways, contests, and more!

 Get exclusive excerpts from our latest releases and videos from *Hay House Present Moments*.

 Enjoy uplifting personal stories, how-to articles, and healing advice, along with videos and empowering quotes, within *Heal Your Life*.

 Have an inspirational story to tell and a passion for writing? Sharpen your writing skills with insider tips from *Your Writing Life*.

Sign Up Now!

Get inspired, educate yourself, get a complimentary gift, and share the wisdom!

http://www.hayhouse.com/newsletters.php

Visit www.hayhouse.com to sign up today!

 HAY HOUSE

 radio for your soul™

HealYourLife.com ♥

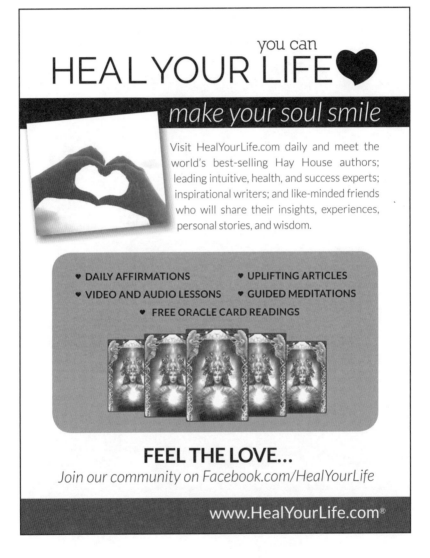